The Commodity
of CARE

Politics and Poor Nursing Care

CAROL DIMON (and *tim*)

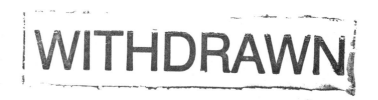

D1470704

The Cloister House Press

First published in the United Kingdom in 2013
by The Cloister House Press

ISBN 978–1–909465-11-4

This book is dedicated to Barbara Robb, and others who have raised issues of standards of care, and to any patients and staff who have suffered within the system.

About the author: Carol Dimon is an RGN, university lecturer, independent researcher, and author. Believing that patients' needs and wishes are paramount, for many years she has raised issues of standards of care at a national level.

Contents

Glossary   ix
Acknowledgements   xi

Introduction   1

1 Historical perspective   7
  The historical effect of the Protestant Work Ethic on nursing

2 Research and campaigns   10
  The ineffectiveness of nursing research and initiatives

3 Care homes within the UK, USA, and Australia   24
  Poor care and the impact of privatisation

4 Hospitals   35
  Poor care and the impact of privatisation

5 Attitudes to care   42
  The effect of the focus on individualism

6 Intellectualisation of care   50
  The end degree level nursing?

7 Poor care and the Care Quality Commission   58
  Ineffectiveness as a regulator

8 Care in the balance   59
  A UNISON survey of staff/patient ratios

9 The issue of remuneration   61
  Nursing pay and morale

10 Truth about welfare spending   63
   Facts and figures

11 Regulation of healthcare assistants
   Government opposition   67

12 Whistleblowing   69
   Repercussions of reporting poor care

13 Ombudsman   73
    Types and effectiveness

14 Failure of the Nursing and Midwifery Council   78
    Areas of failure

15 Human rights and discrimination   83
    The ineffectiveness of legislation

16 Dilemmas of care   88
    Covert nursing practice

17 The exploitation of overseas nurses   90

18 Conclusion and further recommendations   92

    References   96

Glossary

ACAS	Advisory, Conciliation and Arbitration Service
ACB	Anti-Corruption Bureau
ANA	American Nurses' Association
CHRE	Council For Healthcare Regulatory Excellence
CSV	Community Service Volunteers
CQC	Care Quality Commission
DH	Department of Health
ECCA	English Community Care Association
EU	European Union
EUR	Euro
FIR	First Information Report
FT	Foundation Trust
GCSE	General Certificate of Secondary Education
GDP	Gross Domestic Product
GMC	General Medical Council
GNVQ	General National Vocational Qualification
GPC	General Practice Consortia
HCA	Healthcare Assistant
HSCA	Health and Social Care Act 2012
ICN	International Council of Nurses
IELTS	British Council's International English Language Testing System
LGO	Local Government Ombudsman
LHW	Local Healthwatch
NASUWT	National Association of Schoolmasters Union of Women Teachers
NAVCA	National Association for Voluntary and Community Action
NHS	National Health Service
NMC	Nursing and Midwifery Council
OECD	Organisation For Economic Co-operation and Development
PCT	Primary Care Trust (replaced by GPC)
PEG	Percutaneous endoscopic gastrostomy

PHSO   Parliamentary and Health Service Ombudsman
PM   Prime Minister
PSA (formerly HRE) Professional Standards Authority for Health and Social Care
RCN   Royal College of Nursing
RN   Registered Nurse
Rs   Rupees
RUHS   Rajasthan University of Health Sciences (India)
SEK   Swedish krona
USD   United States dollar

Acknowledgements

We wish to acknowledge the following:

Amnesty, who emailed me a copy of the Rights Act, Australia.

Anita De Bellis (Australia), for some fantastic work, and references, including Ronalds. She also emailed me her complete PhD. We need more of such liaison.

Eileen Chubb, from *compassionincare*, who allowed me to publish her content.

GMC, for their emailed response.

ICN, who replied to me regarding their role.

i@independent, who gave me links for journalism regulations.

MONITOR.

King's Fund Centre, for resources and information.

New York Times, for several links to relevant articles.

Professor Jennifer Matthews (USA), who sent several articles and links, in addition to encouragement.

Anne Melcus (Australia, via Linkedin), for information regarding Australia and University database overseas.

NMC, who replied to some questions, but not to others.

DH, who replied to some questions, but not to others.

FOI Officer: Parliamentary and Health Service Ombudsman.

FOI Officer: Local Government Ombudsman.

My local Relatives and Residents Association, who clarified some information.

My local Head of Adult Services, for clarification of information.

LH.

NHS England.

Professor Alan Pearson (Australia), for offering to assist with information.

Dr Kylie Porritt, who Alan Pearson suggested to assist.

Martha Turner (ANA USA).

Zoanne and Kay Leonard; two allied professionals who raised the issue of bogus universities abroad.

Lynnette Chipp, who checked some of the work.

Cath Shepherd, who read some of the text.

Keiren Robertshaw, graphic designer.

We also thank "the voices" – nurses, student nurses, and care assistants; patients and relatives, who speak out and by doing so give insights into the *realities* of nursing care.

Introduction

The aim of the book was to analyse why *poor nursing care* is still occurring within care homes and hospitals in the UK, the USA, and Australia, despite numerous recommendations over at least 30 years. It became evident through the course of research that provision of care depended on the dominant political ethos, sometimes termed *free market* ideology or *neoliberalism* – terms describing an economic theory which claims *the market* should be the sole determinant of people's lifestyle choices, and that the market should be free from government interference, since it is self-regulating.

This book will document the pervasive influence of some neoliberal reforms of healthcare. The emphasis will be on what negates good nursing care delivered with a compassionate attitude. Any reform, from whatever political perspective, that promotes good, compassionate care should be supported by all nurses, who should equally oppose measures that lead to poor and indifferent care. The many recommendations given over decades in reports of poor nursing care have come to nothing; a fact implicit in the continuous repetition of cases of poor care, both within hospitals and care homes, whoever operates them. These recommendations focused on "making the system better", with suggestions of how nurses should be organised (team nursing, as one example); how nurses should respond to patients as individuals (patient-centred care approaches); how complaints procedures should be more readily available and acted on. Such recommendations did not consider how the dominant political ethos in any society affects standards of nursing care; they attempted to address nursing care as if it existed in a political vacuum. Politics determine the amount of money allotted to nursing care; the way in which this is spent (private versus public provision); and the nature of those undertaking care, for the "cult of self" that has been encouraged in *free market* economies does not lend itself to developing caring and compassionate attitudes toward others, who are sometimes seen as "less deserving", if unemployed, or "burdensome to the young", if old, and needing adequate health funding. Such divisions are crudely exploited by politicians.

This book is politically on the side of the patient, whether in a hospital or private nursing home. This author has not conducted her research in any other political sense, that is, an a priori political view has not been the prism through which all findings have been judged.

This book will consider how the dominant political ethos impacts on care in nursing homes and hospitals in the UK, the USA, and Australia, and similarly influences organisations involved in nursing regulation and education, and attitudes towards care of the elderly. This book will draw upon correspondence with various organisations, and will include the "voices" of those involved in front line care. The need for a complete overall of nurse education and the use of students in a hands-on capacity is one of several radical recommendations given in this book; which should have relevance to all those involved with patient care in the private, public, and voluntary sector.

This book offers a *snapshot* of nursing and the organisations that regulate it in 2013. It is recognised that these organisations are subject to rapid change, and that what is given herein is likely to be superseded in a relatively short time. Yet, although the names of regulatory organisations may change, with some amalgamating, and their area of concerns being more finely tuned, it will not be a difference in type – they will continue to regulate a system based on business models of care provision.

Deregulation, privatization, and withdrawal of the state from many areas of social provision is the new norm. Almost all states have embraced, either voluntarily, or in response to coercive pressures, some version of neoliberal theory, and adjusted policies accordingly. Coercive pressure is reinforced by international financial and trade institutions, such as the World Bank, and World Trade Organisation. Universities have also *internalised* these values to such an extent that neoliberalism is the only accepted paradigm of influence; they are increasingly run on attract-as-many-as-possible business models, with a diminution of academic standards to accommodate mass participation; students are encouraged to obtain higher degrees, which, by them being less scarce, become of less value. This is rather like the upper-deck of the Titanic being crowded with PhD graduates from the lower decks, in a deluded belief this will give them the opportunity to survive.

If markets do not exist in areas such as education and healthcare, they must be created, by state action if necessary. State interventions in markets must be kept to a minimum because, according to the theory, the state cannot possibly operate in the economy better than private business. This definition of neoliberalism was not popular in the West until the early 1980s, with the electoral victories of Ronald Reagan and Margaret Thatcher, who both advocated a series of neoliberal reforms that were heavily influenced by the philosophies of right wing thinkers, Friedrich Hayek and Milton Friedman. Thatcher was driven by a vision of adopting a philosophy of anti-socialist economics – the Government should cut public spending, taxes, and refrain from anything but *light touch* intervention in the economy. Competition is central to these ideas. This philosophy separates the fit from the unfit. People are unequal by nature, but this is an advantage to society because the fittest, in a Darwinian sense, will contribute more to society, which will benefit everyone; the example of 19th. century philanthropy by rich industrialists is often given. Nothing is owed to the weak, the poorly educated, what happens to them is their own fault, not the fault of society.

Furthermore, neoliberalism has infiltrated beyond the institution and into the individual. It has pervasive effects on ways of thought, to the point where it has become incorporated into the way many understand their world: the result of endless streams of propaganda disseminated by the media and unquestioning educational institutions. Thus, the UK government's response to the Francis enquiry (2013), into poor nursing care in Mid Staffordshire NHS Foundation Trust, was wholly predictable – envisage patients as "consumers" going to a supermarket; get them or their relatives to rate the service provided (using nebulous questions that will produce whatever result is desired); then justify the hiving off of failing services to the private sector. Individual "consumers" of nursing services will be expected to pay for their care through private medical insurance and pensions.

The government's rhetoric of empowerment is an example of Orwellian doublespeak, which is saying one thing and meaning another, usually its opposite. When watching the news, ask what is the message they are trying to get me to accept? When you hear "the young should not have to pay for the care of the old", they are preparing you for the sales pitch, i.e. "so the government is enacting a new policy of everyone having a private pension that will pay for their care when old". Everyone will be encouraged to take out private health insurance. Not only are sections of society set against each other, a divide to rule ploy, but the individual is expected to meet their future care costs, irrespective of whether they will be in continuous employment, or of whatever illness may ensue. Care bought by private medical insurance in the USA is discontinued when funds become insufficient to meet the costs of commercial care facilities. Thus, the individual of the future is "empowered" to spend the results of their lifetime of work on a private facility of their choice, probably run by a multi-national corporation, in which government ministers may be shareholders; a choice much diminished by the vast commissions taken by pensioner providers:

"Pension-selling companies are taking the equivalent of 80% of money paid into some pension plans out in fees and commissions, BBC Panorama has found. In one HSBC pension plan, £120,000 paid in over 40 years would result in fees and commissions totalling £99,900. HSBC said it takes a 20% profit margin on the pension through the fee structure. It said it offered "good value for money", and was "certainly not one of the most expensive pension schemes in the market". The Co-Op Individual Personal Pension would take out nearly £96,000 in fees across 40 years of investment growth upon deposits of £120,000. Legal and General's Co-funds Portfolio Pension would take out about £61,000, according to the company. In the City, some experts say high fees risk turning some pensions into what are known as "dog funds", or poorly performing investments" (bbc news, 2010). This situation does not seem to be improving, as commented by David Sharkey: "consistently under-performing fund managers currently control around £23 billion of assets invested by millions of small investors" (edp24.co.uk 2013).

Consider parallels between what is happening to the UK education system: Economic rationalism, in the guise of government interest in school improvement, has led to an intensification of individual accountability, and league tables, which falsely seek to reduce complexity by attaching precise numerical values to ambiguous terms such as strong leadership, which can mean many things, from inspirational to dictatorial. He who sets the question shapes the answer. The government line on education testing is that it is necessary to raise standards, but it actually leads to a dumbing down of learning. The proclaimed rise in attainment of academies is due to a thirteen-fold increase in GNVQ entries; a GNVQ intermediate pass is roughly equivalent to an E in GCSE, but statistically the government regards it as the equivalent of four C-grades (Wrigley 2008). Similarly, there is an ideological motive behind hospital improvement.

This book will show how the *free market system*, embedded within the Protestant Work Ethic, has historically impacted on nursing care, and also show that Darwin's ideas of survival of the fittest have been grossly misused in the justification of modern social policy, as he pointed to a social model of survival, wherein groups adapted to their environment through collaborative rather than individualistic effort.

It is important to acknowledge examples of good care, as qualities of kindness and consideration have always been the hallmark of the majority of nurses, who in many cases are called upon to exercise them in the face of stressful work situations. In a UK care home, a resident had his request met every day for chicken, replicating his diet when at home. An elderly resident in a care home who never had visitors was a member of a certain religion. A nurse visited the local religious establishment to explain the resident's plight; consequently, the resident received six visitors from the *church*. A hospital nurse was concerned about patients in pain who suffered from dementia; she undertook a pain management course, and implemented new assessment methods.

The Protestant Work Ethic, as discussed hereinafter, in its guise as neoliberalism, shapes every aspect of present-day nursing. Countless books and research projects over the last 40 years have repeatedly shown examples of poor care, and have made countless recommendations, yet nothing has changed. Each report of poor care is wrongly seen in isolation, as the result of unique circumstance; take, for example, abuse identified in the Mid Staffordshire enquiry (2013), which was seen as resulting from managers focusing on budgets at the expense of patients. How can nursing care be unaffected by the *marketisation* of the NHS, the growing dominance of private corporations in the provision of public services?

Timoney (2013) suggests: "The shrinking of the public sector is self-consciously defined by (neoliberalists) as a return to the night-watchman state of laissez faire Victorian Britain, but the manner of it looks more like a return to the monopoly corporations and royal warrants of the 17th. and 18th. centuries, with all its attendant corruption and cronyism. Privatisation is essentially enclosure and rent-seeking. As more of its functions are privatised, government loses its capacity to do things and becomes more dependent on commercial agents. This leads to an ever closer identification and overlap between politicians and business people. Party politicians in the post democratic age are obliged to simultaneously admit their powerlessness, accepting that whole swathes of life must be left to the market, while trumpeting their ability to correct market abuse and bring wrongdoers to justice".

He also stated, "Fingers are wagged at amoral bankers and newspaper proprietors, but the end result is the same squalid compromise of self-policing and light-touch regulation".

This author fully endorses the right and duty of anyone involved with patient care to voice their concerns, whilst realising there are repercussions for doing so – "cold-shouldering", with people sitting alone in staff rooms, being given the worst jobs and being denied promotion.

There are different complaints and regulatory bodies within England, Scotland, Northern Ireland and Wales.

1
Historical perspective

The philosophy underpinning delivery of care can greatly determine the type and quality of that care. UK asylums and workhouses aimed to deter individuals from dependency on the state (Rose 1971). Hence, care was not an attractive option. For example, individuals had to wear uniforms, work laboriously for long hours, and were punished for trivial misdemeanours. However, there is evidence of exceptions to such harsh rule (Longmate 1974 in Dimon 2006), depending on who was in charge of the establishment; a case in point concerning 18th century Bedlam: "The rooms were bright and comfortable and the inmates were encouraged to read and occupy themselves quietly. Sophie found Mrs. Nicholson, who had tried to murder George III, reading Shakespeare, and asking for some more quill pens. The man at that time in charge of the asylum was Dr. Monroe, who insisted on fresh air and cleanliness, and that the patients should be treated kindly" (Bayne Powell 1951).

In 1789, Vincenzo Chiarugi, superintendent of a mental hospital in Florence introduced regulations providing patients with high standards of hygiene, recreation, and work opportunities; and minimal restraint. Contemporaneously, Jean-Baptiste Pussin, superintendent of a ward for "incurable" mental patients at La Bicetre hospital in Paris, forbade staff to beat patients, and released patients from shackles. Philippe Pinel continued these reforms upon becoming chief physician of La Bicetre's ward for the mentally ill in 1793. Pinel began to keep case histories of patients, and developed the concept of moral treatment, which involved treating patients with sensitivity, and without cruelty or violence. In 1796, a Quaker named William Tuke established the York Retreat in rural England, which became a model of compassionate care, enabling people with mental illnesses to rest, talk about their problems, and work. Eventually these humane principles became widespread in Europe.

Kosciejew (2012), summarised attitudes toward the mentally ill in 18th. and 19th. century North America, having alluded to mental illness being commonly seen as the work of the devil, or God's will: "Some people with mental illnesses received care from their families, but most were jailed or confined in almshouses with the poor and infirm". He mentions the American physician, Benjamin Rush, who brought about change in the Pennsylvania hospital in the 1780's, introducing: "heat and better ventilation in the wards, separation of violent patients from other patients, and programs that offered work, exercise, and recreation to patients".

Following the example of Pinel, institutions were established that catered for the mentally ill; one example being the Quaker-founded Friends Hospital, opened in 1817. Conditions for the majority of poor, mentally ill patients, however, remained poor. Dorothy Dix, a Boston schoolteacher, campaigned to draw attention to their plight, and as a result 32 hospitals were established by 1880. These hospitals soon became overcrowded and understaffed, little more than warehouses for the poor, mentally ill patient. Another campaigner, Clifford Whittingham Beers, brought attention to this in his book A Mind That Found Itself (1908), which detailed his experiences as a mentally ill patient. Beers founded the National Committee for Mental Hygiene, which promoted humane treatment of the mentally ill. The Clifford Beers Foundation was established as a UK charity in 1996 to promote mental health (cliffordbeersfoundation.co.uk).

Hitchcock et al. (londonlives.org), discuss factors shaping the care of the ill in the UK: "With the growth of associational charities in the eighteenth century, several Voluntary hospitals were founded by philanthropic men who wished to ameliorate the lives of the poor, contribute to the increasing population and prosperity of the nation, and improve their own social position. The criteria for admission to these hospitals varied, but it was never automatic. Hospitals rarely admitted those with contagious diseases, and many prevented entry to those with venereal disease, or charged higher fees. Only the two royal hospitals and Guy's accepted fever patients, and only Guy's and the Middlesex admitted incurable patients." These authors show that: "Admission typically required some combination of nomination by a governor or subscriber, a petition, the payment of fees, and provision of a surety who guaranteed to pay the burial expenses if the patient died ... Most hospital patients were from the lower classes as wealthier Londoners preferred to pay doctors to attend to them in their homes ... Reflecting the broader functions of hospitals at the time, as well as the reforming zeal of some of the founders, patients were often subjected to attempts at moral and spiritual care as well as medical cure. Patients were expected to work and receive religious instruction. Those at the London Hospital were required to thank the Hospital Committee on their discharge and go to their parish church to thank God for their cure. Rules prevented patients from leaving hospitals without a pass, and punished those caught swearing and cursing, drinking, stealing, and behaving immodestly".

The Protestant Work Ethic, with its emphasis on individual redemption through work, and individual responsibility of contributing to society through work, is the prevailing ethos that effected attitudes toward treatment of the ill, and is still prevalent.

2

Research and campaigns

Another example of a prevailing ethos (of a care delivery type) was the medical model of care, a term first coined by Szasz in 1961, in relation to psychiatry, and involves treatment according to a medical diagnosis, with professional dominance and exclusion of the individual from decision making (Scullion 2009). The same approach is evident in hospitals, care homes, and other areas of care (Scott 2010). However, use of the medical model is supported by some authors and practitioners, who argue that the patient can be involved (Shah, Mountain 2007).

Another ethos effecting care is institutionalisation (Goffman 1961), in which, as a consequence of staff dominance of patients, there is routine provision of care, such as toilet rounds, regardless of a patient's individual needs or wishes. This may be considered by some to be an efficient (i.e. cost-effective) method of care provision. British P.M. David Cameron wants nurses to focus on "patients not paperwork" while all hospitals will be expected to implement regular ward rounds "to systematically and routinely check that patients are comfortable, are properly fed and hydrated" (Topping 2012). Although this is not a call to reintroduce wholesale task orientation, it does place a ward round (task) as central to good care. The RCN supports the idea: Patricia Marquis, regional director of the RCN south east, said: "We are in support of the announcement and keen to see it happen. Nurses by and large came into the profession to care for people. But over a long period of time this has slipped away. A lot of time is taken up with paperwork and collecting information and data" (portsmouth.co.uk 2012).

Jocelyn Cornwell (2012) wrote: "Active nursing rounds – variously known as "intentional" or "care and comfort" rounds – are still relatively new. What is important is that it is patient rather than task-focused: Every hour, a nurse checks in with the patient, not to *do something to her*, but to find out if she is comfortable and if there is anything she needs. It started in the United States and has been adopted in some UK hospitals". (An article, "Effects of nursing rounds on patients" (Meade, C., et al. 2006, American Journal of Nursing), highlighted a study on hourly rounding as a nursing best practice in hospitals across the USA). Cornwell continued: "One of the problems with the Prime Minister's announcement is that it implies nursing rounds are the solution to poor-quality care everywhere. It is not. It is relevant to some – but not all – wards. It will not compensate for inadequate staffing and it will not work where there are not enough qualified nurses on the ward. But we do know that quality is not completely dependent on resources, and that poor care does happen on adequately staffed wards. But where there are enough staff, nursing rounds can ensure that nurses deliver a reliable standard of care to every patient. Skill mix is another ingredient for success. Having adequate support staff to partner with registered nurses by making rounds on alternate hours is crucial, otherwise nurses will be taxed if they are expected to make rounds every hour".

"Some nurses lack the fundamental attitudes to care", a senior nurse has warned, and said the situation will not be tolerated. It comes after damning reports by the Patients Association, and healthcare regulators, the CQC, that found a series of nursing failures, including patients on hospital wards being left in their own excrement, drinking from flower vases due to thirst, left in pain, and ignored by staff. David Cameron has ordered a review of nursing care, saying he wanted to see hourly ward rounds to make sure patients are comfortable, after being told of "chilling examples" of poor treatment. NHS London, which oversees healthcare in the capital, has ordered universities to implement higher standards on nursing courses. The move followed concerns from senior nurses in London about poor standards of literacy, numeracy, and poor attitudes towards patient care among some new students" (Smith, 2012). The possibility of hourly rounds (concentrating on task orientation) on wards with severe shortages of staff is, as Cornwall suggests, highly problematic. Staff may also refuse to deviate from rounds, or sit at the desk in between rounds (anecdotal). Yet, research does indicate improvements achieved by regular ward rounds, such as reassurance of the patient (Dean 2012). Such rounds, at least, would ensure that every patient sees and communicates with somebody on a regular basis.

A total emphasis on task orientation may detrimentally affect staff, reducing their morale, and preventing them from thinking about the quality of the care they provide. It may reduce stress for some in this way (Menzies 1980), but may increase it for others, contributing to staff burnout (Heine 1986). Responses are dependent on individual characteristics and ways of coping, as indicated by Schimizutani et al. (2008). The concept of personality types may explain differing levels of job satisfaction among nurses working in the same environment. They may also influence a continuation of poor care as a norm, with nurses and care staff conforming to the example set by dominant individuals. In the majority of real life situations conformity is the norm. People go along with the crowd so as not to be ridiculed or ostracised.

The strength of desire to conform is a personality trait whereby some people will try to conform to whatever group they are in at the time, whilst other 'non-conformists' will go in the other direction, deliberately asserting their individuality by rejecting all but a very few sets of norms (Asch 1951). According to the studies by Maslach, Santee, and Wade (1987), part of the masculine gender role is to be independent and assertive, therefore leading males to conform less. At the same time, they stated that part of the feminine role involves being sensitive to others, therefore leading to conformity to maintain harmony. These contrasting personality traits found in men and women set a solid foundation for their conforming or nonconforming behaviours. Cultural differences may also determine levels of conformity. Collectivist cultures (such as the Philippines) conform more because nonconformity is associated with deviance (Kim & Markus, 1999). Western cultures have more individualist attitudes, thus, people from those cultures are less likely in general to conform. Research shows average conformity rates in collectivist cultures of between 25% and 58%, whereas in individualist cultures these rates are between 14% and 39% (Smith & Bond, 1993).

Evidence from criminology further supports the case for gender differences being implicit in degrees of conformity, with women being more reliant on group (gang) membership (Steffensmeier, Allan 1996).

It is recommended that managers of care homes and hospital wards consider the composition of their nursing teams in terms of personality traits, so that dominant types do not impose a conformity of poor care.

Blog voices:

Concerns over hourly ward rounds are echoed in USA blogs from 2009/2010: "No matter the unrealistic expectations placed on a R.N. by administration a prudent nurse prioritizes her time and skill and delivers care to the patients according to acuity and safety. The truth is we do far more than we are ever able to document. Hourly rounding documentation may be needed to prove patients are being checked on but it is not a true reflection of care given. It is nurse/patient ratio that improves care if in fact administration is concerned with improving care at all".

"I work on a 36 bed med teaching floor. We typically have a ratio of 9 patients per RN, with only one or two aides on the floor. Hourly rounding sounds great on paper, but putting it to practice is a joke … The 90 year old dementia patients are constantly checked on because they usually have no concept of time and will call the moment you leave the room. Nurse's discretion dictates that those that need more care receive it. With a mountain of charting and admissions to do and only one aide to help out, realistically, that's the way it's got to be. If administration wants me to recite my script every hour to these patients and sign my sheet, they need to mandate a better nurse/patient ratio".

"I have done hourly rounding for about 2 years and I have not seen the success from it to be honest. Patients call whenever they want something and don't wait until you come back. The numbers at our facility support my viewpoint, call lights didn't change much and patient's are still falling. The patients that constantly call out and are at risk of falling don't grasp the concept of hourly rounding and therefore will still push the button constantly and still climb out of bed. The answer is not only hourly rounding, but better nurse/patient ratios" (blogs.com/medscape).

The ward round as a central nursing task is also going back to the days nurses existed for patients' needs, however menial, and their job was to fulfil them. This was overseen by a sister, who was usually very authoritative, but neoliberal cultural changes have made such authority a negative constraint which undermines individual freedom, and neoliberal influence in fostering a cult of self has not cultivated caring attitudes that no amount of ticking boxes will replace. In fact, the hourly ward round may be nothing more than a paper exercise completed so that a ward can pass an audit. There are many elderly patients who cannot express their needs; will their care needs be properly met, especially at night, when staffing levels are particularly low, or will a box be ticked to suggest they have? What of the nursing home resident? The majority of elderly care in the UK, USA, and Australia takes place in privately run care homes. Such businesses are unlikely to be over-regulated by governments of neoliberal tendency.

Comments by Dowbiggin (2012) support some elements of institutional care: "Most think that criticism of institutions is a recent thing, born out of the 1960s counter-cultural attacks on traditional society. At the time, Thomas Szasz, Erving Goffman, Michel Foucault and others vilified mental hospitals as "total institutions," where inmates allegedly endured lives of ritual abuse or callous neglect ... families came to appreciate them as a means of public welfare, a place to house a relative or friend who simply couldn't be cared for at home. Whether kin had a nervous breakdown, threw destructive and violent fits, or developed dementia, the asylum appeared to be the best alternative for families at their wit's end ... Then governments launched the deinstitutionalization movement. All of a sudden, the experts were proclaiming that people with mental disabilities did better in the community, where they could lead more independent lives. This theory of normalization soon reigned supreme, but theory and reality proved to be two very different things. People with mental disabilities repeatedly fell through the cracks of the system, and ended up on the street, unmedicated and vulnerable to both the elements and crooks who preyed on them".

There have been attempts to oppose task orientation approaches, especially since the 1980's; one such being *primary nursing*, introduced by Alan Pearson, at Burford, 1992, which involves the registered nurse being responsible for 2 patients, with an associate nurse being responsible when the primary nurse is not at work. This demands a higher number of qualified nurses. An alternative is the *key worker system*, which has been used in some care homes. Some versions of this involve the care assistant having specific responsibility for a number of residents, involving tidying wardrobes, or ensuring they have adequate toiletries, etc. There are also such approaches as the Eden alternative, which was proposed in the USA in 1991, and now is used in other countries, including the UK and Australia. This approach involves a culture change in nursing homes, and is based on ten Eden principles, focusing on promoting development and growth of the patient, and a more satisfactory quality of working life of staff (Edenalternative).

In 1977, three experimental NHS nursing homes were established (Graham 1983). These were based upon a Danish approach which involved more person-centred care, such as providing residents with individual letter boxes, setting up residents' committees, and showing respect by knocking on residents' doors. These initiatives enabled residents to feel empowered (Bond, Bond 1996), but were closed down to a lack of funding.

In the 1980s, nursing development units were introduced into the UK, funded by the Kings Fund centre (Wright 2001). They were also introduced in other countries, such as Australia. Their aim was to promote education and research to promote practice based on patient-centred care. The units tried to share good practice by arranging open days, and producing publications.

Nursing, *in theory*, has moved towards person-centred care, with Government emphasis upon this in some countries (McCance et al. 2011); where the patient is the focus, and their wishes are considered. For example, if a patient does not want to get out of bed, they must have sufficient information to make that decision, and be aware of all possible consequences, such as pressure sores (Dimon 2006). Forcing patients to comply to care could be detrimental to their health (Seligman 1975, Dubree and Vogelpohl 1980, Tuckett 2006). Person-centred care is sometimes termed humanistic or holistic (Shi, Singh 2003).

The *humanisation* of care has been written about by authors for many years (Howard, Strauss 1975). Certain nursing models do consider the patient's wishes to a greater extent than the medical model, such as King's model (King 1971). Yet, the value of nursing models is debated (Littlejohn 2002). Does a nurse apply one model at all times to all patients? – as if all individuals are a homogeneous psychological entity. "In nursing, models are often designed by theory authors to depict the beliefs in their theory" (Lancaster and Lancaster 1981, cit. currentnursing.com 2012). They provide an overview of the thinking behind the theory, and may demonstrate how theory can be introduced into practice through specific methods of assessment. Models are useful as they allow the concepts in nursing theory to be successfully applied to nursing practice (ibid.). Their main limitation is that they are only as accurate or useful as the underlying theory. Peplau's concepts of health, as an example, implies "forward movement of the personality and human processes toward creative, constructive, productive, personal, and community living" (1992); the idea that someone needs to work (be productive) in order to live a fulfilling life is a central tenet of the Protestant Work Ethic. Like attitudes effecting care, nursing models cannot be seen in a vacuum – they reflect the social norms in which they exist (Hardy 1986). The current dominant ethos, neo-liberalism, which embraces elements of the Protestant Work Ethic, places an emphasis on cost-cutting, and this imperative constrains the implementation of humanistic models of care more than countless research articles and campaigns promote it.

There have been numerous campaigns in the UK to promote better care: Dignity in Care campaign (Dept of Health), and the CARE campaign (2013), involving the RCN and the Patients Association, are examples. Voluntary bodies are also leading campaigns for better care: The Alzheimer's Society promote Putting Care Right. The Royal College of Psychiatrists runs the Partners in Care Campaign. The National Care Forum exists to promote care and research in care homes. There are also campaigns in Australia and the USA. Better care initiatives are not new: Robb led a campaign to improve care in the UK. In her book, Sans Everything (1967), she wrote (preface x) that: "Staff in institutions develop neurotic self propagating traditions such as misplaced loyalty of one staff member to another. Only a deviant will shop a colleague ... senior staff develop misplaced loyalty to committees ... To criticise forcibly rather than to cover up is to rock the boat. Victimisation of anyone who is critical, whether justifiably or not, may be automatic. Poor references, bad ward assignation ... no promotion, are some of the more obvious punishments". Robb's observations are as pertinent today as when they were written, as are the accounts of contributors to her book regarding staff shortages, one such, Sister Laura Heneage writing: "Mrs. Kingsway died soon afterwards. On the day of her death, there were only myself and Nurse Cavendish on duty. We had neither an orderly or ward maid. We finished breakfasts at 9 a.m. Nurse did beds by herself. I did medicines, saw to dispensary and doctors. By that time it was 10.30 a.m. I made and served coffees, which took me to 11a.m. Various patients were requested for X-rays, etc., and by 12 noon we had not attended to Mrs. Kingsway. Noon to 1 p.m we served dinners. The patient died at 2.40 p.m ... she had not received any attention from my going on at 8 a.m to leaving at 1 p.m". Robb recommended a stronger complaints procedure, with improvements in education, and small institutions, such as flatlets. Her report, based on comments from staff and patients, was regarded as being unreliable (Martin 1984), yet it was based on thousands of replies from staff, patients and relatives to a published letter; It did, however, result in an investigation.

In 1984, Martin analysed major incidents within UK hospitals concerning older people, mentally ill, and mentally handicapped people. A major finding was an inadequate complaints system, with the suppression of complaints by managers and the Government, and absence of follow up of inquiries. Recommendations included staff training, improved management and staff support, improved complaints procedure, staff levels, and care centred on the patient. Unions were described as focusing more on union solidarity than professional criteria. The question is, why were earlier attempts disregarded?

There have also been several Government attempts such as Essence of Care (2010), 1st Created (2001), with aims to improve standards across the UK within the NHS (Department of Health 2010). Has anything fundamentally changed?

Hunter (2012), a relative of an elderly patient in Australia, states: "She probably wouldn't have survived her time in rehab or respite had it not been for mum and I noticing complications that developed while she was in care. There is no question in my mind that the dangerous cellulites in her legs would have remained unnoticed by the medical staff charged with looking after her, at least until it was beyond treatment with antibiotics".

Responding to care that is of poor quality, where care practices are problematic, but do not meet the definition of reportable abuse, is not so straightforward. Given the extent of reportable abuse, it is reasonable to expect that witnessing poor quality care might not be a rare occurrence. Examples of such care practices include those that are not responsive to individual resident preferences or requests, long delays for care, and lack of compassion.

Krause (2011) found that over 30% of U.S. nursing homes were cited for an abuse violation during inspections between January 1, 1999 and January 1, 2001 (U.S. House of Representatives, 2001). The report also found that over 9% of all U.S. nursing homes during that period were cited for abuse violations that caused actual harm or placed residents in immediate jeopardy. The actual prevalence of nursing home resident abuse is likely even higher due to underreporting (Hawes, 2003;

McCool, Jogerst, Daly, & Zu, 2009; Peduzzi, Watzlaf, Rohrer, & Rubinstein, 1997, in Krause 2011). Due to the widespread nature of abuse of nursing home residents (Hawes, in Krause 2011), there is potential for researchers to directly observe or indirectly learn of resident abuse while conducting research in nursing homes.

Responding to care that is of poor quality, where care practices are problematic, but do not meet the definition of reportable abuse, is not so straightforward. Given the extent of reportable abuse, it is reasonable to expect that witnessing poor quality care might not be a rare occurrence. Examples of such care practices include those that are not responsive to individual resident preferences or requests, long delays for care, and lack of compassion.

Krause tells of a nurse researcher who conducted a study about certified nursing assistant (CNA) work in long-term care, and had already interviewed several CNAs, and was in the process of conducting field work. The field work consisted of spending several shifts shadowing and being 'schooled' by the CNAs about what it was like to work in the nursing home.

During this shift, the CNA began speaking quite harshly to a new resident. She told the man, sharply, to "roll over" so she could pull a sheet out from under him, then turned to the researcher and described how this resident had soiled himself. The man, who was evidently very embarrassed, began to cry. The nurse researcher noted that the door to his room was open and that several staff in the hallway, including the nursing supervisor and the charge nurse, overheard the CNA. A few looked in her direction. The charge nurse and nurse supervisor looked over at her, listening to what she was saying. However, when the CNA was finished, the nursing supervisor resumed her conversation with the charge nurse as if nothing unusual had happened. Believing that this incident did not fit the state's definition of reportable abuse, the researcher was uncertain of the best way to proceed.

According to some USA state laws, the above example would clearly meet the definition of reportable (verbal) abuse, and the appropriate response in that situation would have been for the researcher to report her observations to the appropriate state agency. However, under other state laws, the CNA's actions would not have constituted reportable resident abuse, even though those actions were highly problematic. Are we concentrating on research, and the promotion of an academic view of caring, at the expense of real human values?

Based on interviews and literature review with the aim of examining public policy and nursing homes, Vladeck (1980) discusses a lack of privacy and dignity in USA nursing homes, with the over-sedation of residents being one example of poor care. He writes of unskilled staff, and a high staff turnover. Vladeck (p. 213) concludes: "The generally low quality of nursing home care and the apparent indifference to it reflects attitudes towards recipients of public welfare and the institutions in which they live". Bennett (1980) became a nursing home resident for 10 days, and was formerly an administrator of a nursing home. The home manager was aware. Whilst ethics and subjectivity of evidence are questionable, he identified such issues as isolation of residents from the community, and restricted decision-making of residents, with staff who were reluctant to take risks. Revisiting the issue, Vladeck (2003) refers to a newspaper article (Pear 2002) describing abuse in nursing homes, stating: "not enough seems to have changed over the last 25 years". Recently, DeForge (2011) shows some care homes in Canada being places where regular physical abuse occurred. An allnurses.com blog mentioned nurses who sat at a desk and refused to answer call bells (2012). Such blogs are not to be ignored, as journals will not publish everything.

In the UK, Wade et al. (1983) explored care of older people in longstay hospitals, nursing homes, and the community. Morris (1969) undertook research in hospitals and nursing homes, and found that homes were less regimented than hospitals, but identified factors including staff shortages. Wells (1980), in a study of care of older people in hospital, writes of "depersonalised and routine care". Clough (1981), writing about care homes, discusses residents forced to walk, woken at 6.30am, and individual wishes being ignored. Townsend (1962) also refers to lack of choice within nursing homes and other institutions. He recommended increasing community care, thus reducing the need for institutions.

As early as 1966, dehumanisation was being described in institutions for the mentally ill in the USA (Vail 1966). Diamond (1992) worked as a nursing assistant in a USA nursing home and wrote about cold showers and restraint. Newton (1979) kept a diary as a nursing home patient in Australia and wrote of issues such as rigid rules and lack of visitors. Tulloch (1975) was a resident in a USA nursing home and discusses lack of choice and inappropriate staff attitudes. Gubrium et al. (1975) undertook research in a USA nursing home, and found over-use of medication to quieten patients, and waking patients at 5.30am. Laird (1982) was a USA nursing home resident, and spoke of rigid rules and "dehumanizing care".

Amber Paley (2012) reports on abuse in UK, USA, and Australian care facilities: "In the US, the Department for Health and Human Services found that 91 percent of nursing homes fail to meet federal requirements for care. Seventeen percent of nursing homes between 2005 and 2007 were reported for exposing residents to abuse or neglect that did or could have resulted in serious injury. In 2004 alone, more than 500,000 cases of elder abuse were reported in the U.S. She reports on one particularly harrowing case: "One particular story that hit home with many Americans in 2011 involved ... a 78 year-old resident of the Quadrangle Senior Living Community in Haverford, Pennsylvania. Sensing abuse, McCallister's daughter and son-in-law placed a hidden camera in her bedroom. What they found was horrifying. A dementia patient, the video captured McCallister being hit, taunted, poked in the eyes, and having her ears pulled. According to the court affidavit during the majority of the 12-minute encounter recorded by the camera, McCallister stood naked from the waist up attempting to cover her breasts". Abusers were not always care workers: "More than 60 percent of abusers of the elderly were a family member and 13 percent reported their abuser as a care worker. Additionally, women were found to be more likely to suffer from abuse than men; 3.8 percent of women surveyed reported abuse while only 1.1 percent of men did".

Paley continues: "Other harrowing cases of abuse have happened in Australia: In 2010, the story of Gwendoline Gleeson, an 89 year-old patient at Ballabill House Nursing Home in Seymour, Australia, died of a coronary while physically restrained on a toilet. Gleeson, whose health had been deteriorating, had been restrained without medical authorization. Even worse, when her son was told of her death, he was not told the full details; Her son told ABC News: What I heard today from the Coroner's Court was that Mum was strapped in the toilet and she was left there for two hours ... I had never heard of that before". Paley states that cases like these are "not uncommon", and that there is "no established agency that works to truly comprehend elder abuse's prevalence ... According to the USA's National Center on Elder Abuse (NCEA), only 1 out of every 14 cases of elder abuse is reported". Paley suggests: "citizens must take action by spreading the word, creating or joining organizations that educate and act to end abuse, and encouraging politicians to take action". Yet, whilst these sentiments are fully supported by this author, poor care has been reported for decades in the countries mentioned above; there have been numerous clarion cries for action, yet the problem only becomes visible when particularly nasty cases of abuse attract media coverage; there follows a shaking of heads and much talk about the need for action, yet, in that cases of abuse are a continuous feature, sufficient action as not been implemented.

Lee-Treweek (1991) explored the hidden work of the care assistant within two UK nursing homes, concerning the care given within residents' bedrooms. She writes: "mistreatment appeared a fairly everyday strategy to get through the work". Some residents were labelled "whiners", and there was a routine, physical focus. Trained staff appeared to be unaware of a focus upon getting the work done at the expense of compassionate care. Such task emphasis may, in some instances, be due to poor staff to patient ratios. Havig et al (2011) concluded that increasing staffing levels alone is not sufficient to raise quality of care, which depended on other factors, such as leadership. This was based on a study in 21 nursing homes in Norway, involving questionnaire, interview, and observation. The CQC (in Robb et al. 2011) also conclude that poor care may still arise when there are adequate staffing levels, as evident from their inspections. The King's Fund (2012) concurred: "Quality is not completely dependent on resources, and poor care does happen on adequately staffed wards".

Mandelstam (2011) used case studies to analyse care within the NHS. The case of Mrs Clara Stokes: "Her daughter recounted how her 84 year-old mother had been admitted in December 2009 to hospital, where she subsequently died, helpless and confused, after a stroke. She was left dehydrated, hungry, and lying in her own faeces for six hours, being ignored by overworked nurses. Her water was left out of reach, and she had not been helped to drink for 16 hours". The hospital apologised. Other cases referred to alarms being out of reach, records of food and fluid intake not being maintained, and nurses sat at the desk. Mandelstam made several recommendations, including reference to government guidelines being ignored; the Ministry of Health and NHS senior managers should be accountable; a need for the CQC to be given more government support and resources; professional regulatory bodies to reinforce the role of the professional nurse; a need for whistleblowing, involvement of the Health and Safety Executive; and police prosecutions for neglect of patients within the NHS, in addition to care homes.

In Australia, De Bellis (2010) undertook a study concerning nursing practice within aged care facilities. She identifies low staff levels, poor understanding of dementia, registered nurses tending to sit in the office, false documentation, and care described as "neglect", including restraint. De Bellis suggests an adequate skill mix and appropriate staff levels. Tuckett (2007) suggests review of policies and consideration of the whole culture of care within nursing homes in Australia, with "a shift towards the emphasis of effective care and communication". Diamond (1992), writing of USA nursing homes, recommends stronger residents' councils.

Clark et al. (2010) discuss issues of poor care within Australian hospitals, including poor record keeping and excess task-orientation. Ronalds (1989) undertook a study concerning resident's rights in nursing homes and hostels, which indicated excess use of routine care. Woogara (2005) identified that there is little privacy on Australian hospital wards concerning such aspects as sleeping. Tuckett (2005) discusses "production line" care, nurses remaining at the nurse station, and not talking to patients.

Lucero et al. (2009) based on research involving a questionnaire returned by 42,000 nurses in American hospitals, discuss USA hospitals with uncompleted care due to lack of time involving uncompleted care plans and failure to talk to patients. The authors also highlight differences in overall quality between hospitals.

Harrington (2001) details concerns in the USA residential home sector, and concluded: "The story of long term care in the United States holds lessons for the United Kingdom. Because the market is increasingly dominated by profit making corporate providers, the government must be prepared to intervene in areas that affect profit margins and must also retain control over the expenditures of providers in the areas of staffing, skill mix, training, and services provided. Failure to do this leaves regulation in the realm of symbolism and vulnerable, frail elderly people at risk of serious harm". He writes of fewer nurses and lower quality of care with profit-making nursing homes, and notes that low staffing levels are a fundamental cause.

If every care facility had its own independent inspectorate, drawn from its local community, including patient's relatives, who had the legal right to enter a care facility at any hour, and to observe care being given, or care that has obviously not been given, and an obligation to report any instance of substantive poor care to the police, then at least a clear signal will be given as to how seriously society views care of the vulnerable.

The local inspectorate could be given the responsibility of checking on care given within family settings; this would, as in the case of care facilities, provoke outcries of invasion of privacy, and, yes, the majority of care within the family will be good, as it will be in the majority of care facilities; yet to attempt to curtail the abuse of the minority, those who do care should accept such impositions for the greater good; if they do not, then they do not care in a general sense.

Such suggestions will be termed *Stalinist*, and some private care businesses, and some individuals, would oppose them, but if there is nothing to hide, then why?

What was the point of any of such research and recommendations? Their sheer repetitiveness over decades is tantamount to their ineffectuality to change care for the better. They have been substantively ignored by politicians: "Andy Burnham and Alan Johnson, two former Health Secretaries, turned down dozens of requests for public inquiries into the Mid Staffordshire scandal, including 20 from fellow MPs. The Department of Health was handed three reports raising concerns about the quality of care in some parts of the NHS in 2008. The reports by Lord Darzi, a former health minister, found targets were being met at the expense of patient treatment, and identified a culture of fear among staff afraid to raise concerns. These documents were only made public in 2010 as a result of a freedom of information request by Policy Exchange, a think-tank. Andrew Lansley, the former Conservative Health Secretary, announced a public inquiry into the Mid Staffordshire scandal the month after the Coalition came to power" (Mason 2013). Thus, an emphasis is placed on the individual to report poor care, not on the government to fund an adequate number of staff to deliver it.

3
Care homes

In the UK, nursing and residential homes are now all referred to as care homes, and are divided into categories of health or social care, determining whether a nursing home or residential home is appropriate. However, the misplacement of residents into either type of home occurs, with a resident who needs nursing care, for example, living in a residential home. This is often due to funding issues (residential homes usually being a cheaper option than nursing ones), or ineffective assessment procedures; yet, generally, residents in care homes are described as being more dependent than their residential counterparts (Lievesley et al. 2011). Inappropriate placements may affect the type of care that is provided. It is suggested that there is, consequently, a return to a medical model of care, with patients being seen as a task to perform, rather than as a person with individual needs (ibid.). Some homes may be dual registered, which may add to issues surrounding the resident-mix, with residents with dementia disturbing the peace of others through noisy outbursts, invading their personal space, or taking up the majority of nursing staff time.

Some individuals may rather live at home, but are unable to care for themselves. Some may rather live with relatives, but relatives are unable to care for them. Life with a group of strangers is very different from life alone, or with close family, requiring much adjustment (Sigman 2009). Some authors identify a number of stages that are involved in adjustment (Brooke 1989).

For some residents, a care home may signify the end of the road. Fear of anonymity, anxiety, rejection, loneliness, and worthlessness can have a devastating effect on the individual's emotional well-being and ability to adapt to their new life in a care home. Yet, for a small percentage of residents (the less ill) they can offer a new opportunity; consider, for example, the care home residents in the USA who produced works of art (Foundation For Quality Care 2013).

There is evidence of conflict regarding the care home manager's role and budgetary matters (Dimon 2005, Cheek et al. 2013). This may particularly occur within some privately owned homes, in which the manager may remain in the office, occupied with budget and work rota considerations, but they are needed to monitor care outside the office, which may also motivate staff, and to challenge staff about any issue of poor care, which every nurse in the U.K. has a duty to do, according to NMC guidelines (2008). The registered manager has overall responsibility for care, but there may be a regional manager, if the home is company owned, who may enforce budget restraint on the home manager.

It should be a statutory requirement that a registered care home manager should be the main decision maker regarding issues that impact on patient care, such as staffing levels, with the manager being legally obliged to contact nursing agencies in response to poor staff/patient ratios, including emergency nursing agencies. The care home manager should also have a legal responsibility to ensure provision of such things as adequate diets and laundry services, and inform the CQC if standards are not being met, having first raised the issue with higher management or owners. Such an obligation should be extended to managers of hospital wards.

Whilst care homes do have policies, they are only specific to that home, or group of homes. One example of variation was shown in a CQC review (2012), which found: "30% of nursing homes included in the review did not have a 'Do Not Attempt Resuscitation' (DNAR) policy in place (in settings where having a DNAR policy was appropriate and required). Where DNAR policies were in place, most staff (76% of staff in nursing homes) were aware of the policy, although very few (37% of staff in nursing homes) had received formal training in the policy".

Whilst all care homes in the UK are now registered and inspected by the CQC, the past history of care homes and hospitals may have influenced their practices. For example, care homes were previously inspected by CSCI under the CS Act (2000), which placed different requirements on them, such as room sizes (Department of Health 2010).

Care homes in the UK may be owned by the NHS, voluntary bodies, private individuals, or companies. There are still a few Local authority owned residential homes. There are also retirement communities in the UK, for example, the Joseph Rowntree facility in York. Some individuals may actually choose to reside in care homes, paying for their own care, often for the company of others; a problem of endemic proportions, as outlined in a Daily Telegraph report: "Five million elderly people only have television for company as they see friends and family less than once a month, the Health Secretary Jeremy Hunt has said, as he announced new measures for councils to tackle the problem. Surveys will be sent to elderly people and their carers asking them if they are lonely and feel socially isolated. Councils can then offer services such as day centres and meals on wheels where necessary" (Smith 2011).

In the USA, Government agencies, such as Medicare and Medicaid, regulate nursing homes. The USA government has sponsored these important health programs since the 1960s. The Medicaid system provides health benefits to certain low-income groups. The Medicare system provides comprehensive health benefits to those older than 65. Both programs generate strong feelings. Some may feel resentment toward the Medicaid system for any number of reasons, mostly relating to a belief that these individuals have not earned the right to access a system paid by taxpayers' dollars and ,thus, do not deserve it. This reluctance to help the less fortunate, especially if there also is a perception of not pulling their weight, is a telling example of the Protestant Work Ethic and its belief in reward for hard work. There are also additional regulatory agencies per state (Shi, Singh 2003). The USA has Board and Care Homes for those not requiring nursing assistance, which are usually privately paid for. There are also assisted living facilities for individuals who need help with such aspects as medication. Retirement communities enable residents to move between different levels of care on the one site (Shi, Singh 2003). USA nursing homes have also been affected by changes to regulations, such as the Nursing Home Reform Act, 1983 (Formato 2002).

Australia has high and low level care homes (Tuckett 2006). Low level care is deemed sufficient when the individual needs personal rather than nursing care. There are also Ageing in Place homes for both types of care (Australian Government Department of Health and Ageing 2002). In Australia, only 25% of nursing homes are privately owned (bmartin nd); the rest are owned by the Government, or not-for-profit agencies. In the USA (2012), 935 out of 17,0000 nursing homes are owned by private agencies (Wikinvest 2012). In Australia, care standards and an Accreditation Agency were established by the Aged Care Act (1997). These standards also refer to hostels (Weiner et al 2007), which are homes for older people providing low level care.

"All animals are equal, but some are more equal than others" (Orwell 1951). In Australia, Squires (2010) reported that The Sunday Telegraph reporters saw: "Frail residents incapable of feeding themselves left to negotiate often cold, unappetising meals or left to go hungry. Overworked carers ignoring pleas for help to eat, provide blankets or help residents to the toilet or change incontinence pads. Patients left sitting in soaking pads, uncleaned for hours, or humiliated when not helped to the toilet quickly. Severe lapses in hygiene where staff rush between patients without cleaning hands. One worker handling a resident's head while wearing rubber gloves donned to clean toilets. Immobile residents routinely left alone and forced to fend for themselves. Emergency alarm buttons deliberately left out of reach of bed-bound residents. Pleas for medical help following falls ignored, brushed off by busy carers who struggle to meet the demands of difficult patients. Workers ordered to keep families in the dark about conditions, in the homes, including injuries. Elderly residents with overgrown and yellow toenails. Troublesome residents, suffering dementia or other mental illness, heavily medicated to make them more manageable. The Sunday Telegraph also witnessed moments of intense hostility, and at times violence, among patients. There were several examples of hostile interaction between residents and carers. The majority of carers are migrants with a poor grasp of English and unable to communicate effectively with patients". This report was based on undercover visits to 2 nursing homes in Australia owned by major private companies.

Kawam (2012) comments on the neoliberal influence on young nursing home residents in the USA in relation to Medicaid: "Part of the reason for this reportedly insufficient care is due to the overriding neoliberal ethic in the United States healthcare system. These young individuals herein called "young nursing home residents" are frequently covered by Medicaid, which scholars have found is guided by the principals of individualism, cost containment, efficiency over effectiveness, and most recently privatization (Boehm, 2005; Hiranandani, 2011). It is posited here that these principals are in direct contradiction with what is in the best interests of the resident for their long-term health and overall quality of life".

Medicaid was enacted in 1965 as part of the Social Security Act, which intended to provide healthcare for those who met specific eligibility criteria (Holahan et al., 2009). Theoretically speaking, it would appear that Medicaid would provide infrastructure for stable healthcare coverage. Kawam notes: "A recent study using government databases to identify contradictions and implications of Medicaid policy, found that, since the Bush Administration's Deficit Reduction Act of 2005, states have been given increasing flexibility in the application of Medicaid (Coughlin, Zuckerman, 2008). This has led to states changing enrolment guidelines; some states have expanded enrolment while others have capped it completely (ibid.). Additionally, this increase in state flexibility is tied to increased privatization as well as overall cuts to program funding" (ibid.).

Voluntary health programmes are accessed by 14 million people a year in the USA; 40% of whom do not have health insurance (Isaacs, Jellinek 2007). A large number of these people are immigrants. Receptionists, physiotherapists, and doctors work for free in such programmes. However, the number of doctors volunteering is reducing, due to time and financial pressures. Medications may be donated, and other services provided, such as X-ray, dental care (ibid.).

In a similar vein to Kawam, Mel Grey (2011) reports on the increasing marketisation of care services in Australia. Grey suggests that care services have become "tradable commodities delivered in quasi-markets (Considine, 2001). Services were put out to tender to private providers, with managers expected "to run the sector more like a business ... where continued funding is contingent on the proven delivery of concrete outcomes" (Western, et al., 2007); i.e. a reduction in costs. Grey further suggests that this gives: "nongovernment services a new and important role in service delivery which would change its ethos from one of charity, social justice and compassionate care, to one of business-like efficiency. Many faith-based organisations who joined the Job Network in its early days later withdrew for this very reason".

Horton (2007) claims neoliberals view of the world as a "vast supermarket". Yet, as Horton describes, the disadvantaged cannot "shop" at this supermarket. This reflects the preoccupation of neoliberalism with consumerism and the acquisition of goods, and neglects to address society's caring role. Horton describes the resulting control held by the ruling class, who have "approval and consent of members of society", as "hegemony". As a consequence, those on welfare benefits may be regarded with less compassion, as they are viewed as not contributing towards the wealth of society. The Government may say they are "empowering" individuals to make choices (when buying private health insurance), but their true aim may be abdication of responsibility, and focus on capitalist goals.

Imagine an 80 year old lady in an isolated village "choosing" her GP or care home. If making a wrong choice, the government's response would be: it was your choice – so it is your problem. In Germany, older people can be sent against their wishes to cheaper care homes in Spain, Thailand, or the Czech Republic (Connelly 2012). The author comments that the "EU prevents state insurers from signing contracts but it is likely to change". Use of other countries is fuelled by lack of staff and poor quality of care within German care homes, especially concerning individuals with dementia (ibid.).

"Councils facing squeezed budgets are increasingly looking to move residents to cheaper homes, which often means they are passed "like parcels to alternatives hundreds of miles away", a report by Ruth Lythe (2013) revealed. She adds: "Councils are increasingly seeking to find cheaper care options for residents because of a toxic cocktail of their own budget cuts and spiralling fees at homes" ... "Figures from data firm Laing & Buisson show English councils are paying £480 per week for residential care in 2012 to 2013. By contrast, the average weekly care home cost was between £528 and £623". In essence, families are being asked to meet the discrepancies between funding and care home costs, which suggests the social care system in the UK is not sustainable, as families on low and medium incomes are often not in a position to finance such costs. Passing the elderly around like parcels, to repeat, treats individuals as a commodity; an item, and is "inhumane". The logical extension of this system is for the UK to follow the German lead, and send its poorer citizens to care homes in countries were the costs are as low as possible.

The dominant political ethos that impacts on quality of care is described by Professor John Ashton, who stated that the Health and Social Care Bill (2011), now the Health and Social Care Act (2012), signified the beginnings of privatisation, with a return to "the poor law" for the *undeserving poor*. Dr Ashton was threatened with disciplinary action for his comments. Dr Horton commented: "Every health professional has a duty of care to patients and the public. The notion that raising legitimate questions about the adverse impact of this Government's health reforms can be punished sends a chilling signal about the kind of NHS this government wishes to create" (Journal of Anaesthesia Practice 2012).

"According to a Financial Times analysis, around 13% of care homes in the UK were rated poor or adequate by the industry regulator during the 2009/10 financial year" (O'Murchu 2011). Trends in the care home sector also shifted. Councils tried to meet old people's wishes to stay in their own homes as long as possible rather than be moved into care homes. As a result, occupancy rates declined and the people who did move into care homes were older and sicker and so more expensive to look after. The average stay in a care home is now about nine months. "People's image of a care home is people playing chequers in a conservatory with a cat running around their ankles that's just not what they're like any more, these are sub acute health-care facilities," said an investment banker. Then came austerity: the government cut funding to councils, which in turn cut or froze the fees they paid to care homes. With inflation rising, many operators' costs are rising faster than their revenues. Companies that also have high debt payments or rents to support are under extra strain" (O'Connor 2011). A contributory factor in poor care is that these care homes are paid for by local authorities who get their money from central govern-ment. If the resident or their representative were given the money to provide care directly, then poor care would be punished by people voting with their feet – surely a tenet supported by neoliberalist theory? More recently, the CQC, in a report published Nov. 23, 2012, based on evidence from 13,000 inspections, found that 27% of health and social care providers inspected in the past 12 months were failing to meet minimum standards; common problems include staff shortages (the worst of which were found in private nursing homes, with 23% of those inspected failing to meet the CQC standard); poor medication procedures, and record keeping, failing to ensure patients have enough to eat and drink, and a lack of respect and dignity – including staff speaking to patients in a condescending manner (CQC 2012).

Who owns the care facility may have relevance to the care provided, with a range of policies and procedures leading to different experiences of care; however, the focus should be not on who owns the care facility, a non-profit organisation or a for-profit one, but on the quality of the facility and appropriateness of patient care. If poor quality of care is the issue, legislation should address those problems regardless of ownership, and not limit patient choice of care provision.

Within some care homes there is a failure to document appropriately in care plans whether a patient has had a fall, or seen the doctor (Dimond 2005). 4% of cases dealt with by the NMC concerned inadequate record keeping (NMC 2011). Poor record keeping has occurred for many years (De la Cuesta 1983), for reasons such as lack of time due to low staffing levels (DeForge et al. 2011). Many staff do not read care plans. It is advisable after days off to read them. Not all information is given at verbal handover.

UK nursing home residents need a whole range of medical services, including mental health teams, dietetics, occupational therapy, physiotherapy, podiatry, continence, falls, and tissue viability (dealing with wounds, pressure sores and ulcers). Only 43% of PCTs (now replaced by G.P. consortia) made all of these available to care home residents. Where the services were available, it could take a long time for an elderly person to be seen – sometimes as long as 18 weeks – which could lead to a deterioration in health (Bosley 2012).

There is a high stress level within care (Nichols 1992, Deforge 2011). More support needs to be given to all staff. Stress may adversely affect staff levels. If staff are absent, agencies must be rung as soon as possible, yet some care homes and hospitals will not allow this (Dimon 2005). The issue of nursing homes being run on low staffing levels is highlighted in several anonymous blogs (2010–2013) by relatives who commented on care provided by a major care home provider (mumsnet.com).

relatives' voices:

"They are always short staffed . . . when people want the toilet they are left shouting because they are desperate".

"Everything is done on a shoestring".

"Cleaning was minimal".

"Awful, halved the cleaning staff, got rid of help at meal times, reduced laundry staff hours . . . hardly any clean towels or sheets".

"I have seen so much mental cruelty from carers".

"They get treated as if they were already dead".

"These people are someone's mum or dad".

"My mum was left in wet and soiled clothing".

"Most homes are the same, they need some press exposure to show how awful they are".

"Run on minimum staff levels to keep the budget down ... paperwork is prioritised above care".

"Money grabbing company".

Ford Rojas (2011) reported on CQC inspections that found: "Pensioners are being washed and dressed by night staff in the early hours of the morning because their colleagues on the day shift do not have enough time. Inspectors at one home, alerted by an anonymous tip-off, found at least 15 residents up when they visited before 6am, most of them asleep in armchairs. Inspectors also found that just three night staff were on duty to look after 37 people". Poor care is more prevalent than some nurses would like to admit.

Of course, not all nursing homes attract such comments, including some run by the same company, but such comments are too far from being exceptional.

UK residents do not always choose to live in a place of care. They may be admitted to care homes or hospitals under the terms of the Mental Health Act (1983) if they are at risk of harming themselves or others (Dimon 2006). However, such a situation was contested in the European Court of Human Rights (2004), referred to as the Bournewood case, regarding a patient who was admitted to a psychiatric hospital (Boyle 2010), resulting in the establishment of the Deprivation of Liberty Standards (2009). The Mental Capacity Act (2005) also protects the rights of those who are unable to consent. People may also be admitted to care homes and hospitals against their will (under Section 47 of the National Assistance Act of 1948), when not mentally ill, if they are unable to care for themselves (Dimon 2006). This section of the Act is presently being reconsidered.

In the UK, hospital patients do not have to move to a care home which is not their choice. However, the patient has "no right to occupy an acute care bed indefinitely" (Age UK 2013). Borland (2011) reports that elderly patients are referred to as "bedblockers", and can be given 48 hours notice to leave the hospital by a court order, with the possibility of the patient paying the legal fees. "The idea has come from a 2006 case involving Barnet primary care trust in North London which used a High Court possession order to remove a patient who had been in hospital for three years after being declared fit to go home. The patient was also made to pay £10,000 in legal fees" (ibid.).

Thus, the choice of private nursing homes given to the relative of a "bedblocker" is restricted to those that they can travel to, which are often run by the same company, as independent and small groups of care homes are taken over by monopolies, which, themselves, are not immune from financial pressures. Southern Cross Healthcare was the largest provider of care homes and long-term care beds in the UK, operating 750 care homes, before it announced its impending closure in July 2011. Four Seasons Health Care, which has restructured debts of about £780m, took over 140 homes once operated by Southern Cross. Four Seasons Health Care had debts of £1.5bn, but exchanged half of that to their lenders in the form of shares, with the Royal Bank of Scotland, the largest investor, taking a stake of almost 40% (Syal 2011). *A report by Rupert Steiner (2012) shows that the debt levels of care home monopolies is a major concern*; he writes: "Thousands of elderly Britons face a risky future after it emerged the UK's biggest care home operators have racked up debts of £5 billion. The size of the staggering loans, along with revelations many are linked to offshore firms based as far away as the Cayman Islands, have emerged as part of an investigation into the sector. The study shows the scale of the loans and the web of secrecy surrounding operators which run homes for some of the country's most vulnerable people". He continues: "The study by pressure group Corporate Watch, which holds firms to account, shows three operators that control 800 homes have had their debt marked down as "risky" by agencies that rate the health of firms ... Four Seasons' parent company is based in Guernsey and Jersey – it has debts of £525m. Basing their companies abroad makes keeping track of finances more opaque ... Richard Whittell, author of the report, said: "Not only is there all this debt and financial issues – the structure of all these companies is so complicated with many based offshore it obviously makes it far more difficult for local councils to see what's going on, as well as people living in the homes ... The problems affecting the industry stem from local authorities suffering reduced funding and turning to the private sector to build and run the homes. Around 430,000 disabled and elderly people live in long-term residential care in the UK, but only one in ten are now in council or NHS-run institutions".

What choice do the relatives of NHS "bedblockers" really have when choosing a care home? In many instances, they have a "choice" between care homes run by one or two companies based in offshore tax havens, and effectively controlled by major creditors. In the case of Four Seasons Health Care, its largest creditor is the Royal Bank of Scotland, which is effectively (82%) owned by the British taxpayer (Reuters Feb. 2013). Is this model of hidden nationalisation of the private care home sector the new reality? – a nationalised private sector complementing a national (privatised) health service, both run on business models that place cost-cutting as priority. Care becomes a commodity. The NHS is being "asset stripped"; its profitable parts being put out to tender.

It is recommended that details of individuals or companies (including banks) who own any part of a care home, or group of care homes, be made available to prospective patients and their relatives prior to any admission into the care home.

4
Hospitals

Hospitals in the UK may be run by the NHS, private companies, or voluntary bodies. In UK hospitals, the ward manager is responsible to the nursing officer and hospital manager, and practice is governed by hospital policies. In a hospital, the registered manager is the chief executive (or equivalent), and does not necessarily possess a nursing or medical qualification.

It is a commonly held belief that the UK is the only country with a NHS, yet hospitals in the USA and Australia are owned by the Government, and provide free care. However, such hospitals treat only people who are American or Australian citizens.

Within Australia, between 2009–2010, 736 hospitals out of a total of 1326 were owned by the Government (aihw.gov.au/haag). In the USA, out of 5724 hospitals, 1045 are Government and local Government owned (aha.org 2011).

In the UK there are 2312 NHS hospitals (NHSconfed 2012). 70% of hospital patients in the UK are older people (Campbell 2013). There are proposals to base traditional hospital services, such as physiotherapy, in the community (Dixon, in Campbell 2013). This is a result of the transfer of the budget from PCT's to clinical commissioning groups (G.P. consortia) established by the Health and Social Care Act (2012). It is claimed that health services will reflect local needs assisted by Healthwatch.

"From April 2013, local Healthwatch organisations will build on the knowledge and experiences of existing Local Involvement Networks (LINks) who work together to improve health and social care services in their area" (cqc.org.uk 2013). However, a regulation to the Health Act (2012) states: "It would not be reasonable for local Healthwatch to take part in the "promotion of, or opposition (including the promotion of changes) to the policy which any governmental or public authority proposes to adopt in relation to any matter". The chairman of the National Association of LINks Members, Malcolm Alexander, said the regulations placed "unreasonable limits on the freedom of the community to campaign for legislation and local policies that will improve the quality of care". He added: "The government appears fearful of a proactive public and is denying it the right to challenge effectively" (Calkin, 2013). Thus, the government's "consumer champion" of health and social care is nothing more than a "rubber stamp" of government policy. Local Healthwatch organisations will have the same right as LINks to "Enter and View" care homes. Martin Green, Chief Executive of ECCA, commented: "More clarity and detail is needed as to what exactly might be required of care homes by LHW and on what guidance will be available around the conduct of LHW when visiting homes or requiring information" (ECCA 2012).

Victoria Macdonald (2011) gives a wider view: "The NHS reforms plan to put up to 80 per cent of the budget into the hands of family doctors. This means that primary care trusts, who currently decide what care to buy for patients, will be abolished. GP practices will instead form consortia and they will buy – or commission – the care. She states: "not all GPs will want to run or manage the consortia. This means there is a business opportunity for private companies and already many are lining up to offer their services". A leaked document to Channel 4 revealed how companies and GPs may profit from this; one company "talks about plans for five per cent cost savings from patient budgets, and that the less they spend, the more there is left over to share between them. It even proposes that in three to five years, the overall business should become profitable enough to attract City investors". Macdonald quotes Professor Kieran Walshe as saying said the conflict of interest in this document was 'elephant-sized', and: 'What this document says is that the GPs in a commissioning consortium, which is a public body, would let a contract to manage the money of that consortium to a company – an integrated care organisation – that those GPs themselves part own'.

An (*nhsforsale.info* 2013) article suggests: "Your GP may send you for tests carried out by companies like In-health, who run imaging and pathology. Your GP may refer you to a hospital for surgery – perhaps performed in one of the privately run treatment centres. When you return home you could be cared for by one of the queue of companies who are now taking over the running of community health services right across the country. The reach and influence of the private sector over our healthcare is growing fast". The article lists services that can be operated by profit-led companies in 2013 – GP surgeries. GP Our-of-

Hours services. Walk in centres. Urgent care and minor injury units. Diagnostic services (including pathology and imaging). Maternity care. Advice about which services are commissioned. Decisions about how patients are prioritised. Non-emergency surgery (including treatment centres). Hospitals, including A&E. Community nursing. Up to forty other community services (including podiatry, diabetes, and physiotherapy). Ambulance services. Prison health. Mental health services.

A report (bbc.co.uk, 2013) shows that freedom of information requests reveal an increase in spending on private ambulance services of £5.4m by the South East Coast Ambulance Service, from £1.9m, in 2010/2011, to £7.3m, in 2012/2013. The report quotes Shadow Health Secretary, Andy Burnham, as saying this proves the government have not set limits on its privatisation of the NHS – "it is cost-cutting privatisation at its crudest" … "even the most serious of 999 calls are being handled by ambulances without properly trained staff and equipment". The report quotes the government's view that private ambulances were introduced by the previous (neoliberal) Labour government.

"An investigation has found that, since 2010, private agencies have been paid up to £1,794 per shift to provide the health service with specialist nurses – compared with an average rate of around £212 a day for those on the NHS pay roll" (Donnelly, Moore 2013). The private agency takes at least 20% of the fee. Meanwhile, 17 hospitals were warned for having low staff levels (CQC, in Donnelly, Moore). Does this mean that these hospitals avoided using expensive agency staff? – their failure to have adequate staff levels being driven by fears of exceeding their allocated budget, which (as failing *businesses*) may lead to their privatisation.

The *nhsforsale* article gives an example of cost-cutting following profit-led takeovers: "A month after being awarded the £140 million contract to provide care in Suffolk, including community care, Serco announced that 137 jobs would be cut". The article also reports on the same company's running of "out-of-hours service for Cornwall and the Isles of Scilly" were it "introduced a new IT system in summer 2012 in order to reduce costs … skilled clinicians have been replaced by call-handlers without medical training who follow a computer-generated script to assess patients … the changes led to a fourfold increase in ambulance call-outs … Serco needed to reduce this call-out rate in order to meet performance targets for which it is being paid. A report in the Guardian (January 2013) noted that the call-handlers have been given instructions over how to "stop-the-clock" on a call when the new IT system reaches a screen telling the operator to make a 999 call for an ambulance ... they are "instructed to check the call before allowing the system to continue and call an ambulance ... Serco has been accused of running the service with too few staff. In the weekend 22–23 December 2012, a whistleblower told the Guardian that some patients and doctors trying to call the service abandoned their attempts because they could not get through".

Campbell (2013) reports: "The coalition's NHS could destroy the trust between GPs and their patients by making family doctors responsible for the rationing of treatment, the leader of the medical profession has warned. GPs would be at risk of being seen as "agents of the state" who are implementing government cuts once the historic change in their role takes effect on 1 April, Dr Mark Porter told the Guardian". There will be 211 GP-led clinical commissioning groups in England which are described by Porter as "the new rationers of care".

Foundation Trusts: By 2014 all NHS hospitals are to be registered as Foundation Trusts according to the Health and Social Care Act (2012). This means that the Government is not responsible for how the hospital budget is spent. A report by Ramesh (2012) states: "With demand for healthcare rising and budgets constrained, many of the best-known names in the NHS are spending taxpayers' cash to buy beds from private companies. St George's NHS trust in south London last year spent £3.25m at nearby private hospitals Parkside – ultimately owned by US private equity firm Welsh, Carson, Anderson & Stowe – and BUPA-approved St Anthony's". This is a policy of NHS (taxpayer) investment in private hospitals, with a return on investment being used to offset the NHS budget. Such state investment in the private sector is not always well spent: The CQC found that a fifth of private hospitals involved in mental health, learning disabilities, and substance misuse failed at least one standard overall (Triggle 2012).

"NHS hospitals in bid to treat far more private patients. Healthcare trusts seek big increase in income from private patients, raising fears of two-tier service" (Boffey, 2013). Boffey adds: "The increase in revenues follows the government's controversial decision to allow foundation trusts to earn 49% of their income from treating private patients. They were previously capped at earning about 2% from private sources". The RCN has raised concerns regarding the removal of the private patient income cap and its potential impact on NHS patients.

The private sector does have different complaints procedures and policies. Also, FT's can legally oppose agenda for change which guarantees salary and terms and conditions for most staff, including nurses and healthcare assistants; such opposition has been challenged by unions (Calkin 2012). Could we see more overseas staff employed by FT's as they are sometimes paid less, and will accept poorer terms and conditions (Taylor 2013).

Indeed, there is nothing to stop a private company from running Foundation Trusts, as UNISON suggests (2003). This has huge implications for the type of patient within hospitals, with more *acute* patients being treated than those requiring long-term care.

In an article, 'Charities' silence on government policy is tantamount to collusion', Williams (2013) wrote: "A charity sector reliant on government contracts would find it difficult to criticise government policy – that's the central message of a new report by the Panel on the Independence of the Voluntary Sector, chaired by the former head of Barnardo's, Sir Roger Singleton". She adds: "Sometimes, it's because there are gagging orders in government contracts. It's not a matter of discretion, it's a matter of law. Other times, they self-censor, on the basis that this dance never ends – they will always be bidding for new contracts. The need to be looked on favourably by the UK Border Agency, or the local authority, or the Department for Work and Pensions, will never go away". Thus, when the DH announce: "CSV, Regional Voices, NAVCA and National Voices have launched a new drive called Healthwatch-Communities Involved, to raise awareness amongst local people and community groups and volunteers about how they can play a greater role in shaping their services" (DH 2013). The independence of these and other charities from government influence can be questioned.

Grimes (2013) points to the potential enfranchisement of the NHS, with hospitals to be treated like outlets of a fast food chain: "The HSCA says that the status of "NHS Trust" will be abolished in 2014, so every NHS Trust has to become a FT. Since the passage of the Act last year it has become apparent that some 60 NHS Trusts will not make this deadline, so the government has extended the deadline to 2016 and trusts who do not achieve this will either close or be franchised to a private company like Circle Holdings (as in the case of Hinchingbrooke NHS Trust)". Grimes continues: "As of 2012, 43 FTs had a private patient unit – separate units within a hospital which only admit fee-paying patients – and the 2012 Forward Plans indicate that 12 more trusts say that they intend to create one. Again, the direction of travel seems clear". Thus, those who can afford it will be given greater opportunity to jump the NHS queue, no doubt encouraged by advertising campaigns targeting them as "winners", as opposed to "losers" who have failed the Protestant Work Ethic test.

Care homes and hospitals seek the cheapest option, by reducing or cutting physiotherapy and occupational therapy services. Such cost-cutting by hospitals is enabled by the Health and Social Care Act (2012), which requires NHS hospitals to be foundation hospitals, with freedom to spend their own budget.

Unused NHS buildings on hospital campuses could be converted by private hotel companies to house elderly people who may have suffered a fall, have dementia, or are waiting for a place in a nursing home. Government minister, Lord Howe, commented: "NHS England would welcome the opportunity to review this model alongside the suite of other potential best practice resources". NHS England is the new body responsible for recommending how local doctors' groups should provide for their patients. These "hotels" would be staffed by "trained carers", and be a cheaper option than nursing a "bedblocker" (Ross 2013). Confused and wandersome patients with dementia would obviously not be suitable for such "hotels", for they would have to be locked in their rooms. What level of training will the "hotel" carers have? Will they be overseas staff working for the minimum wage, who come from a different culture from those they care for? Will the bedridden dementia patient be the recipient of a hourly ward round? This is not to make a political point against private care per se, it is to suggest that many elderly awaiting admission to a care home have significant care needs, and the central issue is how well these needs would be met in these so called "hotels", which would only be that in name. It is totally disingenuous to suggest that they would offer a hotel-like experience as enjoyed by a holiday-maker. Ideological supporters of such schemes are able to make informed choices. Many "guests" in such "hotels" would not be able to. The "hotels" would be run on strict cost-cutting lines, with minimum staff, and trained nursing assistance being on-call. The dignity of patients depends on the quality of care given, and a sufficient number of those providing that care being caring people. Another factor to consider about this suggestion is that, once patients are "parked" in such "hotels", it would be very tempting on cost grounds to keep them there, rather than send them to a more expensive nursing home. Are would-be nursing students to provide the care? Laurance (2012) reports on a lack of ethics in the private healthcare sector: "A private hospital which accepts NHS work has instructed its doctors to artificially delay operations on non-paying patients to encourage them to pay fees. The Department of Health last night branded the practice "unacceptable" and pledged to intervene ... Private hospitals receive taxpayer money for treating NHS cases, but can make larger fees if the patients go directly to them for treatment". In the largely privatised USA healthcare system, there are many who cannot afford care. Voluntary health programmes attend to 14 million people a year; 40% of whom do not have health insurance (Isaacs, Jellinek 2007). Volunteer doctors, radiographers, and dentists work in clinics for little or no fee; medications may be donated. What of the future of UK healthcare? The Department of Health (dh.gov.uk, 2012) glowingly reports: "Charities join forces in push for greater people power". Volunteers, we are told, can play a greater part shaping local services. Such rhetoric masks the acceptance of a soup-kitchen system of healthcare for the disadvantaged.

As Kafka wrote (Metamorphosis), it is possible that people will wake up one morning and find that they have changed – from being recipients of charity instead of the NHS. *Change is happening by such degree that its conclusion is not being recognised by many, who are led blindly toward a false, neoliberal panacea.*

5
Attitudes To Care

The Voices:

"I am me" – a service user.

"Believe the patient" – a service user.

"Care has been made into a commodity" (Diamond 1992 p. 112).

"I have feelings and needs like you. And they are just a chore to you" (Kareen King USA).

Some argue that poor care is not solely the result of staff shortages brought about by economic constraints; that poor care is about a lack of caring attitude. Such analysis does not identify the link between the egocentric basis of neoliberal dogma and the selfish attitudes it fosters. Neoliberal economic policies and the cult of self interest they are built on are one and the same thing, producing both shortages of staff, and staff with uncaring attitudes.

Rev. Dr. John C Berry (2012) also makes the observation that wherever care is provided, it is the values of society and the nature of caring that impact on its quality: "To examine the care offered in the independent sector is also instructive for understanding the "crisis of care" in the NHS. Over several years The National Care Standards Commission and Care Quality Commission identified numerous instances of failing care regarding the "very basics of life". Berry quotes Brogden (2001), to state that respect for people diminishes as the age and 'makes them fit for disposal as detritus'. Berry suggests; "A care home culture, with its routine management of death and disposal, may create an atmosphere in which neglect and abuse become easily tolerated, resulting in carers, who may already be ill-trained and poorly qualified, becoming numbed and desensitized and adopting varying degrees of detachment". Examples of this "detachment" are given: "In February 2011, a report entitled Care and compassion? by the Health Service Ombudsman listed complaints about elderly care from many hundreds reaching the office annually. The dismissive attitude of staff to patients featured prominently. This was followed by instances of neglect: "we read of tongues like dried leather, nutrition and hydration ignored, patients squealing with unmanaged pain, pressure sores thriving, call bells out of reach, lack of cleanliness and comfort, multiple unrecorded falls, the unavailability of bathing or showering, weeping wounds not dressed, and an absence of patient monitoring".

Berry points to a cultural determinant of poor care: "such lack of care and respect for the fragile bodies of the elderly in a culture so devoted to personal comfort and costly cosmetic pampering of the body seems especially repugnant". Thus, the "cult of self" is identified as a contributory factor in poor care, yet the UK government, as mentioned previously, use narrow self interest to justify their plans for the younger generation not to be burdened with the care costs of those elderly who should have paid their own way, and if they have not, are undeserving. Central government has doubled management posts in the NHS whilst drastically reducing the number of beds and nursing staff. Berry blames this for: "a prevailing mentality that fails to appreciate the basic needs of the vulnerable elderly", and suggests that "root and branch structural change is required".

Pedro Perez (2011) commented on aspects relevant to this, when responding to a report by the Health Service Ombudsman (UK) concerning the treatment given to the elderly in British Hospitals: "The report recounted several cases of abuse and neglect received by elderly. Among the examples, the report cites the cases of elderly who do not receive food or water for days or who are neglected in his room without receiving the minimum hygienic care over weeks . . . elder abuse is a lack of an ethics of care in the nursing profession. The concept of "ethics of care" . . . focuses the attention in the particularities, the mutual relation with the other, the sympathy and the responsibility. It values not only the formal rules, but other sentimental elements which give sense to interpersonal relations. In this sense, while the ethics of justice has a cognitive sense, the ethics of care gives a main role to the emotions and virtues. Only the promotion of emotions and virtues can provide a humane treatment to ill and elderly. In contrast, the rational calculation of the optimization of resources will lead to commit the abuses. Therefore, it is necessary to promote an ethics of care in the exercise of the profession of nursing".

Jared Diamond, UCLA professor of geography and physiology, in his lecture, Honor or Abandon: Why Does Treatment of the Elderly Vary so Widely Among Human Societies? (2009), as reported by Lin (2010), suggested that declining respect for the elderly in some industrialised societies was a result of Darwinian survival forces represented by a neoliberalist cult of individualism: The idea that it is human nature for parents to make sacrifices for their children and, in turn, for their grown children to sacrifice for their aging parents, turns out to be a "naïve expectation". This assumption, he said, ignores undeniable conflicts of interest between generations. From a common sense perspective, "Parents and children both want a comfortable life – there are limits to the sacrifices that they'll make for each other". And from a Darwinian perspective of natural selection "It may under some circumstances be better for children to abandon or kill their parents and for the parents to abandon or kill their children".

Societies also vary in how much they respect their old people – or don't. In East Asian cultures steeped in a Confucian tradition that places a high value on filial piety, obedience and respect, Diamond said, "it is considered utterly despicable not to take care of your elderly parents". The same goes for Mediterranean cultures, where multigenerational families live together in the same house – in stark contrast to the United States, "where routinely, old people do not live with their children and it's a big hassle to take care of your parents even if you want to do it".

Diamond also suggested: "multigenerational families are becoming a thing of the past in many modern cities in China, Japan and India, where today's young people want privacy, want to go off and have a home of their own". Diamond highlighted, within the USA, a "cult of youth" which emphasises "virtues of independence, individualism and self-reliance, which makes life more difficult for the elderly who lose some of these traits". He further points to the impact of America's Protestant Work Ethic, "which holds that if you're no longer working, you've lost the main value that society places on you".

Do all industrialised societies have to allow "undeniable conflicts of interest between generations" to result in lessening respect for the elderly and a consequential under-funding of their care?, with politicians, as in the UK and USA, deliberately appealing to the young's self interest by claiming it is unfair for them to shoulder the burden. Such arguments deliberately target perceptions of self interest; false perceptions, in that those targeted will one day be cast as burdensome. The alternative is for societies to set priorities that deliver good standards of care, as in the case of Sweden.

"Elderly people represent a growing share of the Swedish population.

Many are in good health and lead active lives, and most live in their own homes. Sweden invests more of its gross domestic product in its elderly than any other country in the world. As a proportion of GDP, Sweden's allocation to elderly care is almost five times the EU average" (Sweden.SE.). Life expectancy in Sweden is among the highest in the world. In 2010, it was 79.1 years for men and 83.2 years for women. Sweden has the second largest proportion of people aged 80 or over among the EU member states, totalling 5.3 percent of the population. Since more and more citizens in this age group are in good health, their care requirements have declined since the 1980s. Most elderly care is funded by municipal taxes and government grants. In 2010, the total cost of elderly care in Sweden was SEK 95.9 billion, (USD 14.0 billion, EUR 10.7 billion) but only 3% of the cost was financed by patient charges. Health care costs paid by the elderly themselves are subsidized and based on specified rate schedules" (Sweden.SE.). Thus, there is no inevitability to a lack of funding.

Council taxes in the UK pay for a fortnightly collection of rubbish by private contractors hired by the local council, and, increasingly, for little else; community facilities such as libraries and sports centres are being closed, roads are left unrepaired for longer periods, so, instead of council tax receipts being directly channelled to government coffers, with smaller percentages of it being returned to local communities, why cannot local tax provide care as in the Swedish model?

This would be true localism, but the truth is that government rhetoric about localism only stretches to the areas they want it to.

Relations between social groups can be seen as relations of power. Those in government give only a partial view of society that serves to legitimate and justify the status quo. If the ruling class manages to maintain its control by gaining the approval and consent of their electorate, then it has achieved hegemony – the achievement of political stability by persuading members of society to accept the political and moral values and beliefs of the ruling class.

"There's no such thing as society" (British Prime Minister, Margaret Thatcher, in Beresford 2011). Beresford compares this statement to those of David Cameron; both declaring individuals who depend upon welfare as "scroungers". The state is said to be "insufficient as a service provider."

This statement betray neoliberal ignorance of sociological perspective: The belief that the concept of society is a myth, and what exists is a collection of individuals, rather than a collective comprised of individuals, is nothing more than semantic contortion – an attempt to avoid the notion of collectiveness. Instead of a society, neoliberalists claim there are groups of individuals, or collections of individuals, yet whenever individuals establish any sort of cooperative relationship, by definition, they form a society, and society exists because group survival is more efficient than individual survival: The survival of a species, in a Darwinian sense, is assured by groups adapting to changes in their environment through collaborative effort – to grow crops, build villages, as examples. In fact, most species practice interdependent social behaviour; queen, drone, and workers bees perform complementary tasks for survival; the colony en masse is a society; divisions of it do not exist independently.

Thus, two opposing concepts are outlined: methodological individualism and methodological holism, the former holding that individual human beings have the ability to choose and act collaboratively; the latter suggesting that groups have behaviours that cannot be understood by reducing them to their individual parts. In this regard, consider a large organisation with thousands of employees. No individual worker possesses the knowledge to perform all tasks; the organisation requires individuals to act in social, giving way. However much individuals are "designed" to pursue self interest, a contentious point in itself, when placed in a co-operative enterprise, they tend to share and collaborate in order to ensure group (and their) survival. Groups accomplish things much more efficiently than individuals. Thus, when a group is faced with a common problem, it makes much more sense to solve it collectively than individually.

Social institutions are not created by individuals, they require group agreement. The free market concept consists of two types of social agreement; workers who act collectively to create a product, such as a degree; and government, which defends the "free market" with force, protects property rights, and regulates by prosecuting fraud, monopolistic abuse, etc. In other words, the market is only free within the parameters that society agrees to. Neoliberalists who believe that the market allows individuals to act freely are misguided, because the market itself is a social institution, based on a social compact.

A point is this: when factors shaping healthcare are vaguely termed a business model, it does not identify specific forces at work – to give more precise definition gives a clear idea of what it is that may be confronted, which, this author suggests, is the deliberate targeting of an individual's sense of uniqueness, encouraging a belief in their success against the odds, and by adopting a negative attitude toward others.

Negative attitudes have been found in a significant number of nursing populations since the 1960s and 1970s, and although the proportion of nurses with pessimistic attitudes appeared to lessen throughout later decades, negative attitudes still exist today. An early study by Wallston et al. (1976) found nurses reacted to a hypothetical, male patient, described to participants as an "alcoholic" with various medical conditions, far more negatively than they did the same hypothetical patient, with the same medical conditions, when he was not described as an "alcoholic". When the patient was described as an "alcoholic," he was perceived as being more unsociable, boring, uncooperative, and unpleasant. Numerous studies throughout the 1980's and 1990's suggest that attitudes may not have changed from those found by Wallston (Bartek et al. 1988).

In the UK, Wighton (2011) analysed NHS hospital complaints pertaining to attitudes of staff: "George Argent was a cheerful man with an easy manner — the former sailor enjoyed nothing more than his daily jaunts into the local village and meeting friends for a Friday pub lunch. But the 81-year-old was scared and humiliated in the weeks leading up to his death. Shouted at and belittled by nurses, the widowed grandfather was scolded for soiling his sheets while suffering from superbug clostridium difficile, and laughed at when he asked for some clean hospital pyjamas". In cases of attitude, individuals may excuse the behaviour or provide an alternative perspective (ibid.).

Nurses attitudes toward patients with dementia were examined in a Swedish study, which reported a worst case scenario of neutral attitude: "The analysis revealed four dimensions, which related to licensed practical nurses' opinions of the patients -an ethical and aesthetic dimension; an ability to understand; an ability to experience; and an ability for social interaction. The results of the study indicated that, on the positive to negative attitude continuum, the nurses' attitudes fell at the positive to neutral end. This is an important finding owing to the personhood perspective, from which it is reasonable to assume that, with a more positive attitude to people with dementia, the prerequisites for person-centred care will improve" (Norbergh et al 2006).

However, the degree of negative attitudes of staff toward patients with dementia is more fully given by Kada et al. (2009), who found: "Significant differences in hope and person-centred attitudes were identified in this study. Nursing assistants, compared with registered nurses ... had significantly lower hope attitudes. Staff over 50 years of age reported significantly lower hope attitudes than those under 40 years of age. Staff with 10 and fewer years of work experience reported significantly lower hope attitudes than those with more than 10 years of experience. Nurses with specialised training in geriatrics, psychiatry or dementia care had significantly higher hope attitudes, compared with nurses without any special training. The person-centred attitude was lower among participants who were over 50 years old, compared with their counterparts under the age of 40".

Thus, a wide range of nurse/assistant attitudes toward patients with dementia is evidenced, and negative attitudes are also to be found in nursing homes, as reported by Brodaty et al. (2003), who found staff members' five most prevalent perceptions of residents with dementia were that they are anxious, have little control over their difficult behaviour, are unpredictable, lonely, and frightened. Although 91% of staff reported that they were happy in their job, a quarter reported that residents provided no job satisfaction. The five satisfaction statements most agreed with were: "The patients/residents at work nearly always receive good care". "It is important to try and enter into the way patients experience what happens to them". "Relatives are given enough information about care and treatment". "I enjoy my current work situation". "Our work organisation is good". There were significant differences between homes in levels of strain related to dementia care that were not accounted for by the level of behavioural disturbance. Conclusions: Nursing home staff tended to perceive residents in more negative than positive ways. Staff were generally satisfied with their work. Factors other than resident behavioural disturbance are important influences in nursing staff strain".

Another perspective is added by Prielipp et al. (2010), who explore malpractice within the field of anaesthesia, such as failure to wash hands, or removing vital monitors before the patient is awake. They suggest that it is due to "normalization of deviance"; that is, acceptance of doing the wrong thing. In other words, standards become lower, and everyone accepts this as normal. Even managers may come to believe that these practices are acceptable. For example, if patients are woken up at 6am it becomes the norm and people are reluctant to question.

DeForge et al. (2011), based on a study of nursing homes in Canada, concluded that staff are compliant. That is, do as expected and dictated by policy thus rendering staff "unable to care". Whilst some degree of compliancy is required, this should not be done without question certainly considering individual patients and situations. Again, this is the skill of the nurse (Dimon 2006). However, they also find that blame is shifted between staff, managers and politicians. All are implicated. It is not about blame; the focus should be about improving care.

Jewkes et al. (1988) explore abuse within South African obstetric units. Based on interviews of staff and patients and participant observation, "widespread sanctioning of the use of abusive practices by midwives" was found; for example, slapping a patient on the thigh as she gave birth in order to make her do as the midwife instructed. Various reasons for such practice are given within this study, such as reluctance of patients to complain, lack of staff, and that culture may influence attitudes. Hence, there may be a need in some instances to instruct foreign nurses and care assistants about the British culture in which they are to practice.

A study found that south Asian and Black Caribbean carers of people with dementia are more likely to perceive their caring role as natural, expected, and virtuous. In contrast, White British people are more likely to hold a "non-traditional" caregiving ideology, deriving little or no reward from such a relationship, and believing their own lives are "put on hold" while they perform caring duties. One south Asian son said: "You know, as Indians, we always look after our parents ... my father looked after me when I was young and he has done lots and lots of things for me so it's my turn to look after him" (Royal College of Psychiatrists 2008).

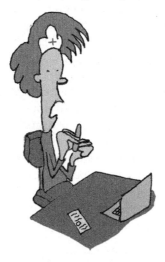

6
Intellectualisation of Care

In the UK, nurses will be required to have a degree from 2013. "The move either escalates nursing to a the lofty intellectual heights it deserves, or condemns patients to wallow in their own filth while the nurses that used to look after them ponder the abstract philosophical principles of post-modern Bauhaus management techniques" (Fleming 2009). A nursing degree student may point out that their course contains ample clinical placement, where practical skills are learned. Yet, what is wrong with having a vocational career? – open to those who would make good, caring nurses? Governments imbued in neoliberalist philosophy will inevitably consider such an option in light of budget considerations, and it is a matter of contention as to whether patient care would suffer. Is the move toward degree level nursing fuelled by the desire of some nurses to elevate the status of their job?

Taking the argument that the prevailing neoliberalist norms of UK politics are not likely to be replaced by a more social doctrine in the near future, the most economic use of nurses as resources would be for nurse training to provide a number of specialist, one year diploma courses, in theatre, acute medical, mental health, etc., rather than a three year degree course, imbued with sociological research, in which students only specialise in its later stages. The diploma courses could involve students learning on the job, as in previous systems of nurse training, whilst assisting with patient care. The education of nursing could be given over to colleges, in which a percentage of lecturers (say, 30%) would be required to be registered nurse practitioners, with at least one lecturer being responsible for overseeing clinical practice, liaising directly with hospitals and nursing homes, to ensure that students are enabled to practice skills in real life situations, and are thoroughly examined in their competency. A single assignment and exam at diploma level would take pressure from students who, at present, struggle to meet the essay-writing demands of their course whilst on their clinical placements.

student voices:

"I am not confident that the training I have received at university is sufficient. Basic skills training is lacking. More time needs to be spent in placement areas and less time essay writing about subjects which have little relevance to a patient's care".

"Yes we need to have academic work but not long essays that stress us out, at the end of the day do our patients really care what grade we get in a 4,000 word essay. I also see some students who are on their final placement that I wouldn't want to nurse any member of my family, and I'm sure the patients think this. Give us longer placements and more practical experience".

"Staff on my general placement thought I was lazy for wanting to spend half an hour talking to patients instead of pretending to work at the nurse's station where I could have read magazines".

"I would love to do basic care, but while on clinical placement we have paperwork that needs to be signed off by a mentor; without which we fail the placement and are not allowed to progress further. On many occasions I have been told by my mentor to stop doing healthcare assistant jobs, and do management work".

"As a third year student nurse I can honestly say that the majority of students do care; maybe a minority who entered training because it seemed a better option than the dole give the rest a bad name".

Ford (2013) reported on a survey of student nurses concerning the government's proposal to establish a one year pre-degree nursing assistant role: a "survey of over 1,400 nursing students found that 42% "agreed" or "strongly agreed" that it was a good idea, while 42% also "disagreed" or "strongly disagreed", saying it was a bad idea. The remaining 16% described themselves as "neutral". When asked whether having to work as an HCA first would have affected their decision to study nursing, 55% said it would not have made a difference and they would have still started their course. 26% said "they might have thought twice" and 19% said they would not have opted not to start their course. Surely, nursing needs to attract recruits from those who thought it a good idea, as opposed to those that disagreed, and who may have entered nursing for reasons other than providing good nursing care delivered with a compassionate attitude.

Such a radical re-appraisal of nurse training will happen, given the internal logic of the market system to cut costs, boost efficiency, get the best value for the tax payer, etc., and this fact will have to be faced by the large number of former nurses who pursued a career in degree lecturing; that their services, like the students they produce, are, in neoliberalist jargon, no longer *value for money*.

nurses' voices:

"I would love to wash a patient, that personal connection is why I came into nursing, but while there are HCA's to do that, I can't justify omitting medications, tests, dressings etc, through lack of time. I hate delegating it to HCA's, when I'd much rather do it myself".

"On my ward they have just replaced four qualified them with 4 HCA's. Now we have an issue with covering sickness, annual leave and maternity with bank or agency qualified staff, who, even if we get them, are not familiar with the ward, so do not know where things are, and, in some cases, cannot speak good English, or perform tasks that you would expect a qualified nurse to be able to do".

"We often run with 2 qualified staff for 30 elderly, high dependant, confused patients. All with complex medical needs. This is with 6 HCA's in the morning, 3 in the evening and 2 at night. The pressure on all staff is unbelievable, and everything now seems to be task focused".

"The lack of qualified nurses on shift and the over use of HCA's who are untrained and poorly paid is largely to blame for what is wrong with the care in hospitals. The ratio of qualified staff to patients is appallingly low in comparison with other countries, who have legal nurse patient ratio's of 1 to 5, whereas we have 1 to 12, or 15 on nights".

"As a nurse I was taught how to assess and check my patients during basic care. This was an opportunity for me to assess nutrition, skin integrity, circulation etc, HCA's are not trained for this and just go in and wash the patient. Because the qualified nurse no longer does this, due to lack of time and management pressure, she misses a vitally important part of her patients care and it's like nursing blindfolded".

"I was a HCA working in acute wards until very recently. I miss the times when you knew you had made a patient more comfortable, when patients thanked you, when you felt like you had made a difference, however small. I don't miss the sense of dread I got during handover. When every single patient, out of 30, needed all cares and I knew that it was just me and the other HCA who had to do it all because the patients were so unwell the qualified would be busy all night with meds, observations, etc. I don't miss finally getting to someone at midnight who had been waiting since 7pm because I had not had a minute until then to help them".

"I have worked in private nursing homes after a career in the NHS, and was recently ashamed to have to say to the nurse I handed over to that I was not allowed by the owners to contact an agency to provide cover for her night shift, leaving her to cope with an appalling staff to patient ratio. If such deliberate neglect were to be repeated in animal welfare then the police would become involved".

"I went to work in a local private care home as my children had left home and I had time on my hands. I was appalled by everything, the food was a monotonous variation of the cheapest mince possible, disguised in various ways, staff were rushed off their feet and had no time to spend with patients, it was like working in a factory. Do people really think that they will not end up in a place like this, that it is them that will be the lucky one? The home was inspected, and the inspection date was known – guess what, more staff and better food on the day".

Nurse educators are charged with preparing pre-registration nursing students to be fit for purpose and fit for practice. In the UK, 50% of students' learning occurs in clinical placements (NMC 2010) where it is expected that mentors will supervise students and provide constructive feedback. However, there have been concerns about the variability of students' skills learning in their clinical placements, which have affected competence levels at registration

Within the UK, whilst the NMC have guidelines which meet EU regulations, the structure of the nursing degree varies per university. Modules are not specified by the NMC (NMC email 2013), but are determined by individual Universities.

NMC standards for education are normally reviewed every 5 years, but feedback is considered from public or professionals. NMC criteria

(2010) identify 4 domains of standards for competence that Universities must address: Professional values, communication and interpersonal skills, nursing practice and decision making, leadership management and teamworking. These domains (standards for competence) must be achieved by the student nurse by the end of the programme. There are a further 10 standards for education, including safeguarding the public, and equality and diversity "which provide the framework for delivery of the programme". Five Essential skills clusters, which address competency of the student nurse (NMC 2010a), include care, compassion, and communication. These factors are to be used as "guidance and incorporated into the programme".

There must be 300 hours of simulated clinical skills (NMC 2010). There is concern about the real value of simulation, which involves dummies in clinical rooms, not real patients. Miskin (2013) suggests that many students lack confidence regarding clinical skills, and do not have sufficient opportunity to practice them in placement. Miskin indicates that effective outcomes may be enhanced by the use of simulation.

The Essential Skills Clusters (NMC 2010b) refer to such practice as PEG feeds. The essential skills cluster of medicine management (number 33) identifies skills to be gained, such as IVI infusions and injections. Other skills are identified (on the second point progression), such as the taking of vital signs. Assessments within practice must be undertaken with the assessment decision made by an appropriately registered person (NMC 2010b standard 8). However, no set assessment method is specified for clinical competency.

It is stated that some clinical skills are not practised by students at all. Curzio, Baille (2009) indicate that 6% of 447 pre-registration nursing a students had not practised measuring BP using electronic or manual equipment when on placement. 425 had attended the simulated teaching session.

Methods of assessment are determined by each University, and may include assessments of simulated practice completed in a clinical teaching room, assessment of essays, portfolios, projects, presentations, and examinations. At least one unseen invigilated exam must be included (NMC 2010b standard 8). The NMC state (2010b) that assessment within the clinical practice area (as well as simulated practice) must be included. The number of attempts a student may have at assessments, is however, determined by the University (NMC 2010b).

Regarding the overall decision of competency of a student nurse, other bodies are involved, such as external examination boards.

The NMC (2006, 2008) recommended a preceptorship of at least 6 months after the student nurses qualifies, to enable them to gain confidence. No guidelines are identified for the content of this preceptorship. Willis (2012) proposed that preceptorship was vital to the development of the nurse. Within the NHS, the Department of Health (2010) require newly qualified nurses and allied professionals to undertake a preceptorship programme. However, the benefits of preceptorship remain debatable (Currie, Watts 2012). Based on literature search, these authors indicate that whilst there are benefits of preceptorship, such as greater confidence of the newly qualified nurses, there is little evaluation of the effect upon quality of patient care, and there are barriers to the process, such as lack of organisational commitment, support or guidance.

Regarding mentorship, when students are on placement there must be a sign-off mentor who has undertaken a programme approved by the NMC, and also a practice-teacher (NMC 2008). The mentor programme must be a minimum of 10 days. There are 8 domains to be achieved by the mentors within their training. The programme must be approved by the NMC, based on 10 broad standards. An ongoing record of achievement must be maintained (NMC 2010b) and evidence of achievements kept by students. At least 40% of the student's time on placement must be supervised (directly or indirectly) by a mentor or practice teacher (NMC 2008).

There are 20,000 student nurses in the UK (Campbell 2013), the majority funded by the Government. The Government (2013) recommends that government funded students spend 12 months working on a ward as a care assistant prior to commencement of their course. This will enable assessment of such skills as compassion. Many oppose this proposal (Guardian 2013), arguing that they may replace care assistants; they may be reluctant to challenge bad practice as they adhere to ward routine, and there may be a lack of mentors. The government suggest that hospitals fund this pre-course training. When hospitals are already under budget pressures, this may well be a proposal that would lead to their "economic" failure, a means to justify privatisation. Other factors include possible repercussions on Higher Education, which will not have an intake of first year nursing students if the process commences universally.

A report commissioned by the RCN, but undertaken independently of them (Willis 2012), suggested there is lack of support for students and mentors on placement. It concludes that a degree is required in order for nurses to practice. It found no evidence that nurse education was directly responsible for poor patient care. This study was based upon responses from nurses and students, and literature search.

The university basis of nurse education is profoundly affected by business models (Popenici, Kerr 2013) that offer the nursing student an academic route leading to a PhD; the student having done little or no actual nursing. The student then finds themselves in competition with numerous others. A weapon of the State is a relentless promotion of positive thinking: "our country must be among the best"; "our country must be a leader"; the individual is encouraged to "persevere and work hard"; "alter their attitude"; "focus their mind". Thus, the problem of unemployment is not of society's making, but one of individual failing. The individual is a pawn in a Lutheran perspective – work hard for personal redemption, and for the good of the state; these aims being synonymous. The student is likewise encouraged to see higher education as a ladder to success; the hard working will progress through the rungs of degrees, to be eventually rewarded with a high status job; a perverse fallacy, as the ever-increasing horde of PhD jobseekers testifies. What, then, is the value of degrees now offered? They are equivalent of painting-by-numbers; the Oxbridge format of balance argument A against argument B, then suggest a compromise, is rigidly imposed, with anything falling outside this format being disregarded. It is format over content, where the mediocre re-create themselves through imposing a mechanics of academia. Education departments try to attract large numbers of students; fuelled by competitive business models. This system is collapsing; students are coming to realise that this particular emperor is naked; his courtiers are propagating a self-preserving myth; it is mass unemployment in the guise of mass education.

Lecturers within this system, nervous of job security, may adhere to delivering safe, non-controversial content to their students, unquestioningly repeating the government's rhetoric concerning plans for people to be forced to be "consumers" in the health market, without analysing what this actually means; without giving alternative viewpoints. Nursing students are being failed at all levels. Too many will never get a job in nursing, having to seek work in a market effected by budgetary restraints and competition from foreign nurses. Some may find work in private nursing homes, but may not be able to cope with the realities of that experience; they certainly would not have been prepared for such realities by their lecturers, few of whom would have experience of working in them, or even have read the numerous reports about them.

When the point comes that neoliberalist governments become less concerned about unemployment among the young, any reason for the present model of education as disguised unemployment becomes defunct, and lecturers within this system will be invited to find alternative jobs.

It is recommended that the content of nurse education be standardised across the UK. A preceptorship for newly trained nurses in both care homes or hospitals should be an NMC requirement, and the content specified. Student nurses should be fully informed of differences between the private sector and the NHS by lecturers who have work experience within these areas.

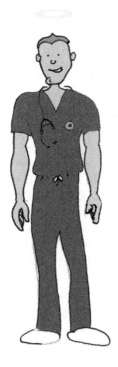

7

Poor care and the care quality commission

The Patients Association (2009) submitted a dossier to the CQC of 16 cases in which it alleged elderly patients were sometimes cruelly treated by staff. Almost all the case histories in the report, Patients Not Numbers, People Not Statistics, come from relatives of patients who died. Many of the allegations were made against nurses, and included a lack of compassion, patients being left lying in faeces and urine, and not receiving the help they need to eat and drink. There were also accusations of mistaken diagnosis, the wrong medication being given, treatment delays, and staff shortages.

There was opposition to the production of the report regarding Mid Staffordshire, led by Heather Wood, of the (then) Healthcare Commission. There were attempts to remove Woods from the investigation by the Health Authority and Strategic Health Authority. Wood commented: "It seemed to us that the top people in the CQC were embarrassed by the Mid Staffordshire report. The leaders of the CQC never had a good word to say about our report. They never promulgated it" (Carvell 2013).

"The CQC has made improvements, including more unannounced inspections, an improved whistleblower helpline, and the employment of additional inspectors (CQC nd)". "Thirty-four care homes and eight agencies providing care in people's homes have closed in the past 12 months (up to Sept. 29, 2010) following regulatory action and the Care Quality Commission (CQC) says the system is about to get tougher. In the same period, another 51 services voluntarily closed after CQC rated them "poor". This includes 39 care homes with about 900 residents, 11 agencies providing care in people's homes and one agency providing nursing care. CQC had demanded these services improve, but had not taken formal enforcement action" (CQC press release 2010).These were CQC's concerns: verbal and psychological abuse of residents, medicines not being managed safely, leaving people at risk of not receiving vital medication, lack of medical and nursing care, staff not legally able to work in the country, poor sanitary conditions, lack of staff training.

8

Care in The Balance

The RCN calls for increased staff levels (Carter 2013). There are no set staff levels in the UK, regulations merely require an appropriate level of staff. Local inspectors may, however, require certain staff levels in care homes; which may be difficult to maintain if staff are off sick, and it is not possible to obtain an agency or bank worker at short notice.

A survey undertaken by UNISON (2012) received 1644 responses, mainly from UNISON members, including nurses, midwives, student nurses, and care assistants, and found that although poor care is a not always due to low staff levels, it is a factor.

A summary of the main points of this survey are that respondents felt – often unable to take breaks or meals due to understaffing and unreasonably high workloads – bank or agency staff don't have the same workplace knowledge as permanent staff, such as where supplies are kept, and so cannot always perform to the same speed or standard as regular staff – unable to report unsafe practices for threat of being bullied or held responsible for the concerns they raised – staffing levels in their workplace impacted directly on the quality of care they were able to provide – the nurse to patient ratio in their workplace on Mar. 6, 2012 was inadequate and that it resulted in the delivery of a lower standard of care – low levels of staffing actively degrades patient care cuts right through the myth that the problem here is with the nursing staff – minimum nurse to patient ratio saves lives and results in better patient care – staff to patient ratios need to be addressed in law, made clear to all and widely implemented – different specialities will require different ratios – high levels of dissatisfaction, stress and frustration.

real voices:

"I am a ward manager and have had nurse to patient ratios enforced on my unit in terms of cost per bed per day rather than the level of dependence of the patients".

"Senior staff change the dependency of patients to suit the number of staff on duty, so as to show that we can 'cope' even when we can't".

"We have set safe staffing levels already. But we rarely run at that level. On the early shift on 6 March we should have had four trained nurses and four healthcare support workers. But instead we only had two healthcare support workers".

"My ward regularly counts students in the numbers".

"12 hours is too long without proper breaks. 12 hours worked, but only paid for 11 hours".

Unison declared: "It is of greatest concern to Unison that healthcare staff are not being afforded their breaks and are being forced to work overtime without pay. Unison understands that sometimes in healthcare it will be necessary to work overtime; if a patient enters a critical condition at 17:40, it won't always be practical for the nurse to pack up and leave at 18:00. This type of overtime stems directly from the healthcare workers' concern for patients. If they left immediately when their contracted hours finished, patient care could be put at risk. Employers are aware of this necessity as well. Refusing to pay overtime for such a commonplace and practical occurrence is placing the employee in a distinctly unfair position. If they stay they will work for free and if they leave they may be putting someone's life at risk. The qualified staff are torn between caring for the patients and the amount of paperwork we have to do, as any paperwork not done has to be finished after shift time ends and we don't get paid for it".

9
The issue of remuneration

Nurses are relatively poorly paid compared to other professions, it is claimed. The basic salary for a typical police officer at entry level is nearly £2,000 more than nurses, teachers and fire fighters, and considerably better than armed forces personnel. Comparisons with nurses and teachers are complicated by differences in benefits, says Charles Cotton in Morgan (2011), who analyses pay and rewards for the Chartered Institute of Personnel and Development. "But you'd have to say that, put next to equivalent emergency personnel such as fire services, the police do seem to be well paid, and even next to the armed forces they do well".

Entry and after 5 year pay levels: Firefighter – £21,157 & £28,199. Police officer – £23,259 & £31,032. Nurse – £21,176 & £25,472. Teacher – £21,588 & £32,200. Soldier – £15,573 & £24,615. Sources: NUT, FBU, RCN, AFPRB, Winsor Review, in Morgan (2011). Hospital nurses' remuneration, ratio to average wage, 2009 (or nearest year) USA 1.3, Australia 1.2, UK 1.1 (OECD Health at a Glance 2011).

Some nurses may point to low remuneration rates as a factor effecting low morale, which may impact on standards of patient care, though pay levels should not be seen in isolation, as Callaghan (2003) concluded: "A large number of nurses were considering leaving the profession and the majority would discourage others from becoming a nurse. The themes that emerged, which related to their disillusionment, included low pay, lack of support for education, limited opportunity for promotion, lack of resources and job insecurity. The findings suggest that while recent salary increases may have helped to improve morale, other factors must also be addressed if further decline in morale and a subsequent nursing shortage is to be avoided".

Odone (2013) wrote: "Almost 8,000 NHS staff earned £100k or more last year. Executives raked in a fortune in the year when an inquiry into the Staffordshire hospital deaths found abuse and negligence was endemic; and when the front-line staff like nurses endured budget cuts and salary freezes. Talk about scandalous behaviour. For a nurse, who takes home as little as £21,000 (less than the national average), this is a slap in the face". Perhaps there is a national indication in all jobs, to reduce the salary paid to the highest earners to lessen the gap. Meanwhile, Foundation Trust hospitals can legally ignore agenda for change (Calkin 2012) which guarantees nurses in the NHS a specific salary and terms and conditions, unlike in the private sector, where staff are generally paid less.

However levels of pay effect morale, as with staff shortages, low morale should not affect attitude whilst care is being delivered, as most nurses would agree, but nurses are also human, and morale is affected by salary freezes and associated financial strains.

Further, nurses and some other staff in NHS are paid according to agenda for change; this does not apply to the private sector. Care assistants within the private sector are generally paid less (McGregor 2011), with many paid the minimum wage. It is disputed whether or not nurses are paid less within the private sector, but, certainly, Agenda for Change does not apply mandatorily. Overseas staff may be paid less both within the private and the NHS sector (Taylor 2012), often accepting the need for experience or training as a reason.

10
Truth about welfare spending

Neoliberal propaganda inculcates the belief that the welfare bill takes up almost all resources, there not being anything left for other projects. This is particularly so in the UK, where such propaganda is repeated by the media to inform the belief system of the indoctrinated. It is important to be aware of the true costs of care, so as to counter such propaganda and better inform people. UK politicians of all shades, that is to say, the same shade with very small variations, tend to lay the blame for the soaring welfare bill on scroungers, and do not mention that 47% of UK benefit spending (£74.22 billion per year goes on state pensions (Rogers 2013).

"The share of benefit spending in gross domestic product (GDP) rose steadily from the late 40s to early 80s, but has since levelled off. In fact, benefit spending in 2011–12 accounted for 10.4% of GDP, less than in the mid-80s or mid-90s. Also, over half of benefit spending goes to pensioners. The state pension, pension credit and winter fuel payments now account for 5.5% of GDP, compared to 4% in 1997 and less than 2% in the early 50s. This reflects less miserly pensions, plus an ageing population" (Gaffney 2012).

(GDP, or Gross Domestic Product, is one the primary indicators used to gauge the health of a country's economy. It represents the total monetary value of all goods and services produced over a specific time period – it can be seen as the size of the economy).

"The most meaningful guide to the cost of the welfare state is to measure welfare payments as a % of GDP. If GDP is rising, we can afford to spend more on welfare payments, without increasing tax rates. Also, between 2001 and 2012, the UK population increased by nearly 5 million. Therefore, the welfare payments per person increased slower than the total welfare bill. This suggests welfare as a % of GDP has stayed reasonably stable at 6% of GDP. There was an increase during the recession – which is to be expected as GDP falls and welfare payments automatically increase. Statistics such as this only show part of the story. To really understand the effectiveness of welfare payments, we need a close examination of each benefit, how it is spent and how it is claimed. It illustrates the importance of being aware of different ways of viewing the same statistics. "Welfare State is out of control as Welfare bill doubles in 10 years!". Alternatively, you could say apart from an expected blip during the recession, welfare payments as % of GDP remain at the same manageable level of 6% .The second headline probably wouldn't sell as many newspapers. But, both statements are based on truth" (Pettinger, 2013).

Total social welfare spending: "Social welfare expenditures are defined as spending for the poor, the unemployed, the disabled, the elderly, and on healthcare. The material reported comes from a historical study comparing the U.S. and the Nordic countries between 1920 and 2003. People's perceptions are driven by the standard statistic reported in the news and in the OECD database: gross public social welfare spending as a percentage of GDP. In 2003, Sweden spent 37% relative to GDP, Denmark 32%, Norway 28%, Finland 26%, and the USA lagged behind at 17%.Yet gross transfers do not take into account the dramatic differences in tax structure in the USA and the Nordic countries. The Nordic countries collect income taxes on the cash payments made to social welfare recipients at rates that are four to five times the rates paid by American recipients. Then when the Nordic recipients go out to make purchases, they pay consumption tax rates on their purchases that are 4 to 5 times the rate paid by the poor in the USA. Furthermore, the USA government offers a series of tax breaks to promote social welfare that are not found in the Nordic countries. After adjusting for the differences in taxation to get net public social spending relative to GDP, Sweden's figure falls by 8 percentage points to 29%, Denmark falls to 24%, Norway to 23% and Finland to 20%. The USA figure rises to 19%" (Price Fishback, 2010).

"The most recent data on social spending in OECD countries shows that in 2007, the year before the global financial crisis, Australia spent 16 per cent of GDP on cash benefits (including pensions and unemployment payments, healthcare and community services) compared to an OECD average of just over 19 per cent" (Whiteford 2011).

Showing latest available data. Weighted averages: 1. Denmark: 29.2. 2. Sweden: 28.9. 3. France: 28.5. 4. Germany: 27.4. 5 Belgium: 27.2. 6 Switzerland: 26.4. 7. Austria: 26. 8. Finland: 24.8. 9. Italy: 24.4. 10. Netherlands: 24.3. 10. Greece: 24.3. 12 Norway: 23.9. 13. Poland: 23. 14. United Kingdom: 21.8. 15. Portugal: 21.1. 16. Luxembourg: 20.8. 17.

Hungary: 20.1. 17. Czech Republic: 20.1. 19. Iceland: 19.8. 20. Spain: 19.6. 21. New Zealand: 18.5. 22 Australia: 18. 23. Slovakia: 17.9. 24. Canada: 17.8. 25. Japan: 16.9. 26. United States: 14.8. 27 Ireland: 13.8. 28 Mexico: 11.8. 29 Korea, South: 6.1. (nationmaster.com 2012).

Spending on healthcare: Another factor that increases cost is poor health-related behaviour of the population. Of course, excessive alcohol consumption, tobacco use and poor exercise increase health problems. The incidence of these behaviours is different country to country.

Many of the countries that spend the most per capita on healthcare have highly privatized systems. In the U.S. and Switzerland, which spend the most and third-most on healthcare, respectively, the government pays less than 65% of the total healthcare costs. In most of the countries in the developed world, public expenditure accounts for at least 70% of total costs.

Many of the countries with the highest expenditure per capita on healthcare also have among the most government-funded healthcare systems. The governments of Denmark, Austria and Luxembourg pay 84% or more of the total healthcare cost. Total public spending in these countries, without accounting for private healthcare spending, ranges from 6.5% of GDP in Luxembourg to the OECD-high 9.8% of GDP in Denmark. In most of the OECD nations, the government foots the majority of the healthcare bill.

"Between 2000 and 2004 the increase in spending on health in the United Kingdom as a percentage of GDP was bigger than the increases in France, Germany, and Italy, says a new report from the Office of Health Economics (OHE). This means that the gap between the UK and other European countries such as Germany and France in total spending on health as a percentage of GDP has narrowed" (Griffin 2007).

Matthews (2009) gave a further breakdown of comparative care costs: "Total spending on healthcare in the UK rose to an estimated £120bn in 2006, representing 9.4% of GDP, up from 7.1% in 2001. Referring to Tony Blair's promise in 2000 to bring NHS funding up to European levels. Of the circa 15% of GDP the US spends on healthcare annually (that's about $2.2 trillion), around 50% is spent by the government (around $1.1 trillion). By contrast, the UK spends around 8% of its GDP on healthcare, with the Department of Health's budget for the NHS (England) in 2008/9 around £94 billion (about $155 billion). The English NHS cares for 49 million people (100% of the population of England); US public healthcare currently covers about 83 million (around 28% of the US population).For a direct comparison, that means that in England the government spends around $3,200 per capita on healthcare and covers the entire population whereas in the US the federal government spends around $3,700 per capita and yet covers less than a third of the population. Take away those 80 million covered by the US's state healthcare (which doesn't cover all uninsured Americans, so this is being generous) from the States' 300 million population, we're left with 220 million Americans to account for the other $1.1 trillion spent in the US each year on private healthcare … that works out as $5000 for every American in the private system – almost $2,000 a year more than the NHS costs … the US free market system for healthcare provision is significantly less efficient than a "socialised" one … you might be tempted at this point to suggest that it is precisely this ability of a national health service to drive down costs that the Republicans are opposed to, as it would leave the rich pharmaceutical companies out of pocket".

It is recommended that the UK spend the equivalent amount on health and social care as France or Germany.

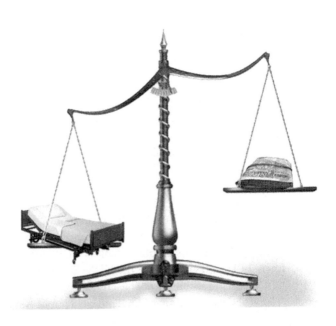

11

Regulation of healthcare assistants

One recommendation of the Francis report (2013) into the Mid Staffordshire enquiry is to register care assistants. If they are registered, it may prevent them from working elsewhere if reported for delivering poor care, but not all cases of poor care are reported, and, If reported, it does not necessarily achieve any action being taken from the manager or registration body (Naish 2012). There is a much larger number of care assistants than nurses, and they mostly work unsupervised. The RCN indicates that there is insufficient training of healthcare assistants within the UK (bbc.co.uk 2011), with care assistants being asked to do far more than they should. This is said to apply to hospitals as well as care homes. The UK Government propose minimum national training standards for support workers in health and social care (Campbell 2013). On March 26, 2013, it became mandatory for NHS establishments to initiate training for healthcare support workers and adult social care workers based on skillsforcare standards (DH) yet how this is done will vary between establishments, although assessment is recorded. The CQC also require this to apply to care homes.

There are reports that poor care is the result of delegating care to healthcare assistants (Collins 2012), who comments: "NHS patients are receiving an "unacceptable" level of care from a growing army of unqualified healthcare assistants who have taken over nursing roles on wards and in care homes, an independent commission warns". This may arise due to the lack of nurses to supervise or instruct them.

Care assistants are not registered in the USA or Australia, but this subject remains under debate.

An NMC commissioned review was published in July 2010 (Griffiths, Robinson 2010), and concluded that the NMC continues to have a central role in initiating action towards healthcare assistant regulation. The researchers found evidence that healthcare assistants are sometimes allowed to undertake tasks for which they are not trained, and that there are cases in which lack of regulation has meant that they have been dismissed from one post for misconduct only to find new employment in a similar role. (In similar fashion, it is possible for a student nurse to fail a fitness for practice panel interview within a UK university, and be terminated from a pre-registration nursing course, and yet still continue in employment as a healthcare assistant (Glasper nd).

"The maltreatment of patients and clients by healthcare professionals and others employed to deliver care features prominently in newspapers, and it seems to be a frequent occurrence. Despite this, it is important to note that Griffiths and Robinson (2010), in their report to the NMC, stress that it has not been possible to demonstrate unequivocally that an unregulated healthcare support workforce presents a risk to public safety, and that this risk would be prevented by regulation" (Glasper nd).

The Government has rejected proposals to register care assistants, considering it would be "burdensome" to introduce and unfair to expect care assistants to pay the registration fee. Yet the majority of healthcare assistants surveyed (British Journal of Healthcare Assistants) would prefer to be registered (Triggle 2013).

12

Whistleblowing

Relatives and patients in hospital or care homes often do not want to complain, for fear of repercussion, or because they are so grateful for any care whatsoever (Ronalds 1989, The Patients Association, in Pickover 2012). Many are unaware of the complaint procedure – this may also apply to some nurses. Many are unaware of the UK charity, Whistleblowers Association, Public Concern at Work, or Patients First. It also takes mental strength and perseverance to complain – the NMC procedure is not easy to follow. There have been fabricated NMC cases that falsely accused nurses who did not *fit in* with their colleagues (Middleton 2012). One way of encouraging a member of staff to leave is to collect minor issues against them.

A recent report by the CHRE – now PSA – (Naish 2012) indicates failings of the NMC. For example, in cases of direct physical abuse of patients, nurses are allowed to continue to practice; the NMC declaring that physical abuse is a matter of attitude and not clinical skill. Of 4407 referrals to the NMC in 2012, only 866 were dealt with by the conduct committee, and 86 by the health committee. This means the rest were closed by the screening committees, for various reasons. Of 650 cases in which fitness to practice was found to be impaired (NMC 2011–2012) in 2012, 365 were removed. Whilst overseas status of individuals is not recorded, such factors as religion and sexual orientation are recorded. Surely, it is more relevant to know where a nurse was trained, so as to identify any factors arising from that training that might lead to them being reported to the NMC Conduct committee.

Eileen Chubb, a former care assistant, (compassionincare 2009) commented on the role of the NMC regards to whistleblowers: 'Of course there were policies and procedures on whistle-blowing in the care home where I worked and they would have protected me had they been stuffed down my clothing as body armour when I was hit in the back with a chair for telling tales, but that was the extent of the protection they offered. I know how many ways there are to make a person's working life a living hell and how much it takes to walk into your place of work and face that hatred until you have no choice but to look for another job, only it does not even end there, I would ring up for a job to be asked, " Are you one of them whistle-blowers from **** home? " and be told the job has just gone. To be left with no job, no money and inevitable hardship as no one wants to employ someone who will speak out against wrong in a care system where so much wrong exists, that is the harsh reality and there is no law to protect you as The Public Interest Disclosure Act is worse than useless. Yes I believe Whistle-blowers should be able to speak out and have so much to say about it have written a book on the subject and have petitioned parliament for better legal protection for whistle-blowers so the government know about all the shortfalls of the current law. The reality is that if you report abuse you as the whistle-blower will be out of a job but the abuser you reported will still have their job as there is no accountability".

Student nurses, in particular, may find challenging poor care very difficult; issues of student nurse conformity to the prevalent norms of their placement has been highlighted in research (Levett-Jones et al 2009), in which students "described how and why they adopted or adapted to the teams and institution's values and norms, rather than challenging them, believing that this would improve their likelihood of acceptance and inclusion by the nursing staff." Yet, nursing lecturers are not required to visit student nurses who are on placement. Universities do, however, have protocols for student nurses to raise concerns, as do NHS and private hospitals, but these protocols involve complaints being kept "in-house", with clauses forbidding "whistleblowers" to go to the press.

One study showed: "Results indicated that there were severe professional reprisals if the nurse reported misconduct, but there were few professional consequences if the nurse remained silent. Official reprisals included demotion (4%), reprimand (11%), and referral to a psychiatrist (9%). Whistleblowers also reported that they received professional reprisals in the form of threats (16%), rejection by peers (14%), pressure to resign (7%), and being treated as a traitor (14%). Ten per cent reported that they felt their career had been halted. These findings suggest that when nurses identify and report misconduct in the workplace, they may experience serious professional consequences" (McDonald, Ahern 2000). The Royal College of Nursing survey (2011) of 3,000 members found a third (34 per cent) had been "discouraged or told directly not to report concerns at their workplace", up from 21 per cent in 2009.

The provision of care is very challenging, due to the many situations which may arise. Nurses are required to be thinking, autonomous, and flexible. These qualities need to be promoted within nurse education. However, students and other individuals may be afraid to challenge others. There may be a reluctance to *whistleblow* due to fear of repercussions (Jackson et al 2010), as reported by Martin (1984).

There is also a lack of support for staff who complain. There have been nurses (Haywood) who have gone to the press or television in desperation (Dimon 2012). Margaret Haywood was removed from the register, but reinstated following petitions, leading to NMC guidelines being revised. Nurses have also been dismissed for complaining in the UK, USA, and Australia (Shifrin 2008, bmartin nd).

There are published reports of people being blocked for reporting poor care. Gary Walker, head of Lincolnshire Hospital Trust was paid to resign (Chapman 2013). Reports include nurses and care assistants leaving the profession altogether, moving elsewhere, or being blocked in career progression.

On March 13, 2013, Jeremy Hunt announced that gagging people is to be stopped immediately (Chapman 2013). £14.7m has been spent over 3 years on 600 compromise agreements with individuals. Whilst he was calling for "openness and transparency", journalists were banned from filming or questioning David Nicholson, who is under scrutiny as NHS chief executive, due to his leadership role in Mid Staffordshire (Chapman 2013).

"A student nurse who exposed the appalling neglect of elderly patients at a hospital trust, where up to 1,200 people died needlessly, has been thrown off her training course. Two years after the Mid Staffordshire scandal, Barbara Allatt reported NHS colleagues for leaving patients in soiled sheets, shouting at dementia sufferers, and secretly slipping sedatives into a cup of tea. But this mature student was condemned for having an "attitude problem", before being withdrawn from her nursing course at Staffordshire University. Miss Allatt, from Cannock, said: "The wards were heartbreaking. There were patients crying out for help but the staff would sit chatting. Some needed urgent pain relief or a change of sheets and others just needed a bit of reassurance, but they were ignored, shouted at or mocked with cruel names. Sick and elderly people were manhandled and abused. But when I complained my colleagues told me to mind my own business. They were so pally with each other that they shut me out and I felt helpless" (Schlesinger 2010).

Within Western Australia, Ahern and Mcdonald (2002) explored the difference between whistleblowers and non-whistleblowers, based on a rating scale. Of significance, they conclude, that the determining factor is the nurse's belief system. Non-whistleblowers adhered to the traditional role of responsibility to the doctor. Whistleblowers were responsible to the patient.

A Nursing Times survey (Ford 2013), which received 847 responses from care staff and nurses, found that 51.7% of the staff who complained had negative consequences; 42.9% would be prepared to raise concerns; 79.6% indicated that the process of raising concerns could be better. Comments received suggested that a greater degree of advice and support is needed, including from the NMC. The degree of support to whistleblowers from unions is questionable (Hart 2013). The RCN was declared as being ineffective by the Francis report (2013), which outlined at least one example of a nurse not being adequately represented when raising concerns of poor care. The RCN is described has having conflicting roles of union and professional body. The RCN is endeavouring to improve their effectiveness (Ford 2013 b), stating that it has "real lessons to learn". There is evidence that unions are weaker than they once were (Milne 2012), due to anti-strike legislation, and their reduced number of members, due to public sector job cuts. Evidence indicates a similar position is in the USA (Economics.about.com). ACAS is a UK government funded arbitration service that represents employees, including nurses and care assistants, by providing advice and mediation.

The RCN's leadership seem more concerned with serving on government committees than representing their rank and file. Whose needs do they serve? "The creatures outside looked from pig to man, and from man to pig, and from pig to man again; but already it was impossible to say which was which" (Orwell 1951).

A further recommendation of the Mid Staffordshire report is to make it a legal requirement for hospital directors to report poor care, termed "the duty of candour" (Francis 2013).This remains under consideration by the Government. Is nobody naturally caring? Will people only care because they fear the consequences if they do not?

In the USA, abuse of patients must be reported by nurses to the manager and Adult Protective Service (Richards 2011). The requirement for reporting errors, such as drug errors, differs per state, and many do not report errors, as they fear repercussions (Robinson Wolf, Hughes nd). In Australia, since 2007, individual care staff must legally report severe, sexual, or physical abuse (Paley 2012).

13

Ombudsman

The Parliamentary and Health Service Ombudsman was established in 1973 (ombudsman.org.uk) to deal with complaints of individuals about the NHS in England. Whilst the CQC regulates hospitals and care homes in England, they will not investigate individual complaints; however, individuals can feedback to them (Pearl 2011). The CQC do investigate complaints regarding issues concerning the Mental Health Act (CQC 2011), and will undertake unannounced inspections based on information they receive (CQC.org.uk). They will also refer people to appropriate organisations, and refer issues to such as Safeguarding Authorities.

Statistics reveal that, in 2012, 16,337 complaints were received by the PHSO, and 150,859 were received by the NHS (Ombudsman 2012). An FOI request (2013) informs us that of 16,337 complaints received, 10,565 did not meet the criteria of the ombudsman, and were reported too soon, or not in writing. 1000 were withdrawn by the complainants. 4399 were "looked at in more detail". Of these 649 were corrected and 400 investigated more fully. This appears to still leave some cases unaccounted for.

Since October 2011, the Local Government Ombudsman will investigate some complaints in England (ibid.). They look at complaints about care of adults within care homes, but they will only consider a complaint once the council or care provider has been given a reasonable opportunity to deal with the situation (lgo.org). Nor will they consider complaints about nursing care; only social care. Yet the difference between social and nursing care is very difficult to distinguish. The Parliamentary and Health Service Ombudsman deals only with complaints about nursing care of NHS funded patients (LGO email), including residents in NHS owned care homes and NHS funded residents in nursing homes.

Regarding the Local Government Ombudsman, in 2011–2012, 20,906 complaints were received concerning all areas of enquiry, such as benefits and education. Of these, 10,627 were forwarded to investigative teams. Of the total complaints and enquiries 2,256 were about adult social care. Of these 1,277 were forwarded to investigative teams (clarified by FOI LGO 2013). The meaning of adult social care refers to all aspects including community care. Some cases were not investigated for various reasons, such as not enough evidence, or lack of power to investigate (lgo.org.uk 2012).

How effective are various Ombudsman? There is evidence that they are powerless and hidden within bureaucracy (Bokhari nd). They are also difficult to access, and not all individuals are aware of them, or the process of accessing them (ibid). In 2011, the UK Health Committee declared that the Ombudsman need to alter their process due to inefficiency: "The Health Committee has found that the role of the Health Service Ombudsman needs a complete overhaul if it is to provide an effective appeals process for the complaints system" (Parliament 2011).

Some blogs indicate a general dissatisfaction with the Ombudsman. There is also evidence of achievement – a report was published by the PHSO regarding quality of care of older people in England, which was very influential (Ombudsman 2011). However, there are reports that the hospitals concerned failed to act against the staff involved (Borland 2011). The ombudsman proposes that the NHS improves its' complaints system, as Julie Mellor stated: "All too often the people who come to us for help are unhappy because of the careless communication, insincere apologies and unclear explanations they've received from the NHS" (Ombudsman 2012).

Further protection in England: When residents in care homes have their fee paid for by the local council, they are represented by a contract between the council's "Contracts Compliance" department and the care home. It has the right to intervene if it suspects that the contract is being contravened by the care home. If serious issues exist, the contract between the council and the care home may be terminated. This is based on the council's standards, of which CQC standards form the basis. Private paying residents may pay via the council, thus also obtaining such cover (local head of adult services).

It is not always easy to find contact details for *Contracts Compliance*, but CQC, local adult services, and local advocacy bodies will assist in this regard.

What is the potential price paid for complaining? UK care homes are within their rights to ask residents to leave at one months' notice, sometimes in response to relatives and residents complaining of care;

with care homes declaring that they "are unable to meet the needs of the residents" (alzheimers.org.uk).

It is difficult to obtain information regarding issues within private hospitals, apart from individual CQC reports There is some evidence that patients are not always informed of the complaints procedure (big-lies.org nd). If the hospital is a member of the Advisory Services, the Association will advise patients and public. If the patient is funded by a private healthcare company, they will advise the patient. Otherwise, the Parliamentary Health Service Ombudsman deals with complaints. "Our claim is that actual numbers of serious untoward incidents in British private hospitals are far greater than publicised cases would suggest, and that this situation will continue until the government finally addresses these problems" (big-lies.org nd).

The complaints procedure for NHS hospitals is given on the NHS website, nhs.uk, which states: "If you are not happy with an NHS services provide you can make a complaint, you should complain to your service provider such as GP, dentist, hospital or pharmacist first. Alternatively, you can complaint to the commissioner of that service. In the past, this was your local primary care trust (PCT). PCTs ceased to exist on April 1, 2013. Now you will have to take your complaint to either the NHS England or your local Clinical Commissioning Group (CCG)". NHS England only considers issues regarding primary care. PALS, within NHS hospitals, will also investigate complaints, which will continue in some manner within FT. There are also local independent advocacy groups linked to the NHS.

In the USA, hospital patients may complain to the Quality Improvement Organisation, regarding medicare, or the Joint Commission, regarding such aspects as rights (Clancy 2008). There are also state hotlines to report abuse (Voldberg nd). There are similar hotlines in the UK and Australia, especially regarding the abuse of older people.

The long-term care Ombudsman in the USA was established in 1972 (aoa.gov 2012) to ensure quality of care and rights for older people in long-term care facilities, such as care homes and hospitals. All states must have a long-term care ombudsman which is independent of the government, and uses volunteers. Individuals are advocates for patients, visit them, and mediate for them (J Matthews).

Other than the older people, there are also several types of healthcare and patient ombudsman (Ziegenfuss 2010), but all vary in type per state.

In Australia, there are Private Health Insurance Ombudsman (phio.org.uk) to address issues regarding private health insurance. Also, there is an aged care complaints investigative scheme re residential or community care, and government subsidised care (Australia.gov.ai Complaints).

There are also healthcare Ombudsman: Australian states have set up services that deal with health and disability service complaints. In South Western Australia "the Health and Disability Services Complaints Office (HaDSCO) is an independent statutory authority providing an impartial resolution service for complaints relating to health or disability services. This service is free and available to all users and providers of health or disability services … Acting impartially and in confidence, HaDSCO reviews and reports on the causes of complaints, undertakes investigations, suggests service improvements and advises service providers about effectively resolving complaints" (hadsco.wa.gov.au).

Medicare and Medicaid in the USA and Australia also provide alternative means of redress. Families tend to use such arbitration services as a given means of resolving issues concerning care. Thus, they are deflected from being critical of the commercialisation of care that has produced these issues; they are not encouraged to question the marketplace system of aged care; they are encouraged to press for more regulation of the system, not the abandonment of it. Emphasis is on complaints mechanisms, unannounced checks, and mandatory reporting of abuse. The focus is on "fixing" a fundamentally flawed system and not fundamentally changing the system.

All NHS patients, including NHS patients in nursing homes, may further approach GPC with complaints, but just how they will be dealt with is unclear (DH 2011). GPC will be responsible for a large percentage of the NHS budget, and will commission many NHS services (Imison et al 2011).

People who receive care from the NHS within primary care from such as dentists and GPs, can also complain to NHS England (england.nhs.uk). Monitor will consider complaints regarding patient choice and competition of services within the NHS, but not health or nursing care (Monitor 2013).

The exact role of Healthwatch regarding complaints depends on how each local Healthwatch define it (National Healthwatch). Some local Healthwatch groups will support relatives and residents making complaints about care homes by referring them to such organisations as the CQC. They may also visit a care home in response to individual complaints.

It can also be reiterated that this book provides a snapshot, as taken in 2013, of those organisations which are charged with overseeing complaints of various kinds, and are subject to change as a result of political decisions.

14

Failure of the Nursing and Midwifery Council

The NMC is failing on "every level and in every system", a review has found. Much of the blame has been placed at the door of the regulator's leaders. Following a review into the NMC, which began in January 2012, the CHRE published its final report (Jul. 3, 2012). Chief Executive and General Secretary of the Royal College of Nursing (RCN) described the CHRE's findings as "concerning" and said many nurses have been losing faith in the NMC for "quite some time". Acting Chief Executive and Registrar of the NMC Jackie Smith apologised for the "substantial failings" highlighted by the review. "The strategic review report and annual performance review report together make difficult reading for the NMC," she said. "They highlight substantial failings in the delivery of our regulatory functions and in the management of our organisation" (Smith 2012).

"Other organisations, such as trade unions and employers, have been recommended by the NMC as "better placed" to carry out an advisory and supportive role" (Nursing In Practice 2012). The NMC's stance seems to be that nurses should self-regulate to maintain the NMC's standards of practice, without the NMC auditing or checking that this self-regulation is actually happening.

Overseas nurse qualifications and the NMC: Overseas nurses were able to register in the UK with the NMC, even with a 20 year gap from nursing (Meikle 2011), and many newly qualified British nurses are unable to obtain work. They may apply for a job on a unit they have worked on, and be told the job has been given to a foreign nurse because the hospital has a contract and a quota to fill for overseas nurses. What is the point of their training if they are not given preference over foreign nurses? Many jobs on the NHS Jobs website are asking for six to 12 months' experience; a difficult thing to obtain if not given the opportunity. There remains a shortage of nurses in the UK (RCN 2013), but this does not take into account unemployed recent graduates.

The NMC do state that they require overseas nurses from outside the

EU to have practiced for 450 hours within the previous 3 years (NMC 2013a) "Research has found that up to a quarter of nurses working in London are foreign, with the largest number coming from the Philippines. Hospitals in the capital that recruit a high number of overseas workers include University College Hospital, the Royal Free, and Guy's and St Thomas" (Telegraph 2010). This factor remains relevant. "Figures show 3,197 nurses from the EU were registered here between November 2010 and November 2011, compared to 2,256 in the same time the year before. Around 87,000 of the 660,000 nurses working in the NHS are from abroad, mainly from the Philippines, Australia, India and South Africa" (Buckland 2012).

Nurse qualifications can also be bought in other countries (Chandra 2012), which may not be identified in the UK, despite checks. There was only one nurses removed by the NMC for falsification of nurse qualification in 2011 (NMC 2012). Any other cases that may have been reported to them, or anybody else, are unknown. There have been cases of people in the UK working as nurses, but not being qualified at all (Williams 2011), due to failure of the hospital to check records with the NMC. Out of 360 nursing colleges in Bangalore in 2003–2004, only 30 were approved (Seekhalakshmi, Soshargiri 2006); a subject given consideration by Parihar (2012), who disturbingly reports of the address of one nursing college in Rajasthan being a vacant plot. Do the NMC check the validity of colleges offering degrees in India or elsewhere? If not, why not? This author has written to the NMC, politicians, PSA, UNISON, ICN, and the DH regarding this issue, and has had no satisfactory reply.

This is also an issue within other countries. Dubai (emirates 2011) discovered 56 doctors and nurses with false qualifications. In Australia, there is a list of approved universities overseas against which qualifications can be validated (Aei.gov.au). The GMC also check Universities against an approved list. Why not the NMC?

Parihir states: "There are 330 private nursing colleges in the state churning out 50,000 graduates annually, 1,000–plus BEd colleges with more than 1,00,000 students and 150 private engineering colleges with 3,000-odd students on their rolls in MTech and 80,000 in BTech. The biggest scam is in nursing colleges. In March, ACB raided 82 of the state's 330 recognised colleges and found that only 10 had the mandatory infrastructure and facilities. ACB lodged FIRs against 21 colleges and initiated a preliminary inquiry against nine others. Some were found to be textile printing units or vacant plots when visited.

Further, there is evidence of payments being made to pass exams; "On May 17, an ACB team caught Surendra Mishra, principal of Upchar College of Nursing, Rajkumari, the warden of the college's hostel, and Ramraj Gujjar, an RUHS clerk, accepting Rs. 20,000 from a third-year student. The student alleged that Mishra demanded Rs.40,000 from her to pass an exam she had failed and threatened to get her failed again if she didn't pay. A cellphone seized from Gujjar had names of nursing students with their roll numbers and names of papers in which marks were to be raised" There is also evidence of exam candidates being given exam questions before the exam (BSc Nursing) within the same article.

This is not to imply that Indian nursing qualifications per se are of questionable standard; this author has worked with many excellent nurses from India, but the larger question of whether the NMC checks the validity of any foreign qualifications needs to be addressed. If they do not, then why are they placing patients at risk, and completely failing in their duty as a regulator of nursing practice?

Based upon an email received from the NMC (March 2013), nurses qualifying within the EU have adaptation training according to their individual needs, which are assessed by the NMC, based on such factors as references, and an outline of their overseas course content. Nurses outside the EU undergo adaptation training of varying duration – 20 days to 9 months. Content is specified by the NMC, and the university courses that supply such training are validated by the NMC.

(Nurses from other countries may be unaware of UK regulations and procedures, such as Deprivation of Liberty Safeguards).

English language testing is to be introduced for doctors (Donnelly, Leach 2013). It was argued that it was against EU regulations to test the English competency of individuals from within the EU, but now the Government realise this was a mistake (Donnelly, Leach 2013).

Those from outside the EU have to provide evidence of IELTS which may be undertaken in their own country. The NMC do require nurses and midwives to be proficient in English, but state they have limited powers to test the skills (NMC 2013b). Donnelly and Leach (2013) state that, in 2012, of the doctors removed from registration by the GMC, 75% were from overseas. Yet the NMC state in an email to this author (2013) that they do not keep such statistics regarding overseas nurses, who now form a huge part of the UK nursing workforce.

All care professionals within France have been tested for many years (Martin 2011). The NMC are reviewing adaptation training, and may now require overseas nurses to attend NMC headquarters with their certificates (NMC 2013b). Fake certificates are difficult to detect – dangers include misunderstandings which can lead to patient deaths. Donnnelly and Leach (2013) discuss the case of an overseas Doctor who gave more than 10 times the recommended dose of morphine. Naish (2012 b) gives an example of a foreign nurse in a care home could not inform a relative what medication the resident was prescribed. Again, the NMC does not record the overseas status of nurses who are convicted at NMC hearings.

Should the NMC have a list of validated nursing colleges in which overseas nurses must have trained, with their fingerprints recorded, so as to eliminate the possibility of fraudulent applications?

A test for EU nurses, regarding paediatric nursing, has been introduced by the NMC, and will be applied to adult nursing and midwives in the future (NMC 2013c). This test must be undertaken at an approved educational establishment within the UK. It is unclear if it will actually replace adaptation training, which, as discussed, is delivered on an individual basis. An email from the NMC to this author (2013) states that it will not replace adaptation training, but nurses "will have a choice of whether to do the test or the adaptation programme".

Does the government actually care about the validity of qualifications, or are they unaware of the real situation? A report by Harrison (2013) concerning unqualified teachers being used as a cost-cutting measure seems to exemplify government attitude: "Last year the government relaxed the rules in England on employing teachers for academies. The semi-independent state schools are now allowed to employ teachers who have not qualified as teachers, bringing them in to line with the situation in free schools and private schools. In other state-funded schools, people employed as teachers have to have passed the relevant qualification – known as Qualified Teacher Status (QTS). At the time, the government said the change would allow schools to bring in talented professionals such as scientists, musicians and university professors, plus experienced teachers and heads from overseas and the independent sector. Schools are also allowed to employ people called "instructors" who have particular – usually vocational – skills but do not have QTS, and the rules governing when they can be hired were relaxed last September. The NASUWT says the changes mean less-qualified people are being put in charge of classes – and are being paid less than teachers. It has published a survey of its members which found six out of ten of those who replied said unqualified staff were being used in their schools and that most said unqualified staff were teaching lessons". How long will it be before that such "flexibility" is allowed within nursing? The inherent logic that drives neoliberalist theory will lead to "talented" individuals being substituted for nurses at lower rates of pay.

"Nursing regulators admit they do not know how many immigrant workers could have fraudulently secured frontline health positions after faking evidence of their qualifications, experience or identity." (McFarlane 2013). From February 2013 the NMC suspended the registration of overseas nurses following concerns raised by some MPs whilst they reviewed NMC procedures. The registration of overseas nurses was resumed on April 2, 2013, but the situation remains under review at this time (NMC 2013b). Changes being considered include requiring all overseas applicants to attend the NMC office with their certificates. Yet how would this ensure the certificates are genuine?

It is recommended that the adaptation training of all overseas nurses is standardised, to address such issues as legislation specific to the UK, within the NHS and the private sector.

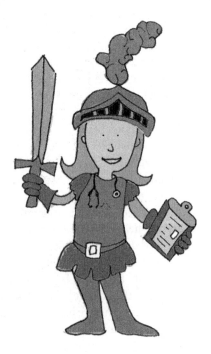

15

Human rights and discrimination

Underpinning the whole process of care is the right of the individual to receive care. If the patient they have no right to receive care, they may not request it, or complain. If the nurse or carer thinks the patient has no right to receive care, they will not provide care, or appropriate care. Some authors suggest that if people are not recognised as deserving of rights, dehumanisation occurs (Vladeck 1980).

What equates to satisfactory care for one person may not be so for another. Individuals have different standards, due to different life experiences. This may explain the lack of general support for some who raise issues of poor care. Some may consider it to be satisfactory for people to be lined up waiting for a bath, for example.

In order to care, it is essential to consider the individual. The dilemma of the carer is to what degree is it possible to do this? For example, how can one individual receive thoughtful and unhurried care amidst a ward of 30 patients? – especially with low staff levels. Thus, an issue of human rights is involved; authors declaring that there is a limit to meeting individual rights when they conflict with the rights of another (Thompson et al 2006). Yet, such philosophical nuance seems to give legitimacy to a status quo that allows, as in the Mid Staffordshire case, elderly patients to be left unattended for hours in a dehydrated and soiled condition. All such patients surely had an equal right to basic care from a sufficient number of conscientious staff. Neither human rights legislation, the plethora of research into instances of bad care, the millions of words written about various models of care, came to the aid of those neglected at Mid Staffordshire; nor do they affect policy on staffing levels that stem from an adherence to cost-cutting ideology.

Patients' rights are an integral component of human rights. They promote and sustain beneficial relationships between patients and healthcare providers. The role of patients' rights, therefore, is to reaffirm fundamental human rights in the healthcare context by according patients humane treatment. The need to protect and promote the dignity, integrity, and respect of all patients is now widely accepted. To this end, the World Health Organization (WHO) predicts that the articulation of patient rights will in turn make people more conscious of their responsibilities when seeking and receiving or providing healthcare, and this will ensure that patient-provider relationships are marked by mutual support and respect (WHO 1994).

In the context of the Human Rights Act, the Alzheimer's Society is especially concerned that the rights of people with dementia are not being respected with regards to Article 3 (right to freedom from torture or inhuman or degrading treatment), Article 8 (right to respect for one's privacy and family life, one's home and correspondence), Article 6 (right to fair and public hearing by an impartial tribunal), and Article 14 (right not to be discriminated against in access to these rights).

In the USA, all healthcare establishments involving Medicare and Medicaid are required to give patients, on admission, information regarding human rights. Some have Bills of Rights (Shi, Singh 2003).In Australia, all care homes possess charters of rights according to the Aged Care Act, 1997. There was a recommendation for this based on a research study concerning residents rights in nursing homes and hostels (Ronalds 1989). In the UK, care homes are not required to possess a charter of rights, but some do have them. Rights are now addressed in the CQC standards for care homes and hospitals.

Would a charter of rights be the ultimate panacea? A charter may merely be an underused document. Also, as noted earlier, patients and their relatives need to know how to complain, and they need support in doing so.

Rights claimed by patients, or permitted by care staff, may be determined by their expectations, or as Tuckett (2005) discusses, their perceptions of what care should be. Tuckett cites the example of a nursing home resident who expected it to be like a medical facility, compared to a resident who expected it to be more like home.

Why might rights of patients be opposed? Several factors may be involved. As discussed, care reflects socio-political factors; within the neoliberal paradigm do "failing" individuals deserve to be cared for?

Bloxham (2011) gave an example of a breach of rights: "Serious failings were uncovered in the care provided to a client named only as Mr J by Northumberland, Tyne and Wear NHS Foundation Trust, Newcastle City Council, and the Coquet Trust. A joint inquiry by the

Health Service and Local Government Ombudsmen found he was kept in hospital unnecessarily for months, and then moved into inappropriate accommodation afterwards. The inquiry found he had day-to-day support from Newcastle City Council, and his family, to whom he was close, supported his wish to be as independent as possible. But when health professionals became concerned about a significant deterioration in his skills and health, Mr J was admitted to hospital for a short assessment. He was diagnosed with dementia and epilepsy but, in spite of being declared ready for discharge, he was kept in hospital for a further five months. Rather than returning home, which was now considered to be unsuitable accommodation, Mr J and his wife were moved to a self-contained flat at a care home for older people. The flat was kept locked to restrict Mr J's access to the outside, for safety reasons. Although this was supposed to be temporary accommodation, Mr J and his wife were still living there 10 months later, when Mr J became ill with a chest infection. He was admitted to hospital, where he died, aged 53. His rights to liberty and family life were not given adequate consideration by those involved in his care, and there was a lack of leadership, the inquiry found."

Such breaches of human rights are not confined to institutions of care. Triggle (BBC 2011) reported on a care review by the Equality and Human Rights Commission (UK), which showed under funding of home care, and also a basic lack of compassion by some of those employed to provide care to vulnerable, elderly people. The review found that basic care for the elderly in their own homes in England is so bad it breaches human rights at times. The home care review by the Equality and Human Rights Commission highlighted cases of physical abuse, theft, neglect, and disregard for privacy and dignity. It said on many occasions support for tasks such as washing and dressing was "dehumanising" and left people "stripped of self-worth".

The findings have added weight to calls for a complete overhaul of the system, yet the for-profit organisations involved in home care will only provide care that protect profits rather than patients, and the pressure on those workers providing home care in the inadequate amount of time allocated for it is unlikely to lessen. There are currently nearly 500,000 people who are getting council-funded support in their own homes. The home care review said about half of people who had given evidence reported real satisfaction with care, but a number of common complaints were made by others. These included: physical abuse; most often in the form of rough handling or unnecessary physical force. A 78-year-old woman who lives alone told the commission about her treatment: "Most of the girls (from the agency) were nasty. They were rough. Rather than say "Sit in the chair", they'd push me back into the chair, that sort of thing, and I didn't like that".

The commission said such problems could be said to be in breach of various parts of the European Convention on Human Rights. Neither private agencies or those they employ are likely to be conversant with European human rights legislation, but this is not the issue; should it require legislation to force those involved in care to act in a humane and respectful manner, for, if it does, then regulatory procedures for selecting those giving care need to be imposed; it cannot be left to profit-making companies to meet their commitments by employing anyone just make up their numbers. Again, is it the case that materialistic society as spawned too many people who simply do not care about others.

The Equality and Human Rights Commission (EHRC) said the law needed extending to clear up a potential loophole. Councils are already covered by the Human Rights Act, but as they buy most home care services from the voluntary and private sector, it remains unclear how well protected the elderly are. But the commission suggested the prospects for the future looked bleak, as one in three councils had already cut back on home care spending, while a further one in five were planning to. EHRC commissioner Baroness Sally Greengross, who led the report, said it was time home care provided by councils was encompassed by the Human Rights Act: "And one of the ways to stop it continuing is to close the loophole, which means that any care that's commissioned by a local authority or another public body should come under the Human Rights Act so people are protected from abuse". As if this would make one jot of difference to the quality of care provided. It is a blinkered and inadequate response on a bureaucratic level, and ignores the indifference shown by some home care workers to those entrusted to their care, which no amount of human rights legislation will impact on. If prosecutions follow proven cases of neglect, a fear of punishment might curtail some bad care, but, again, the real point is missed: why are some people so uncaring? A frightening point also arises: we have no way of knowing what really goes on behind some closed doors and shut curtains.

A further question – is it possible to care for a stranger? Hung (nd) explores this issue with reference to Kafka's "Metamorphosis", suggesting that strangers are people who are different and who we cannot communicate with, hence they are excluded. Wilkinson, Brittman (2003) explore the issue with reference to Noddings (1984), who suggested that we cannot care naturally for strangers. This suggests that some care may be better performed within a family setting, but, as mentioned, many younger people may view a caring role as an imposition on their right to lead an individual-centred life; many would not be able to care for reasons of being employed; some may not even like their parents.

The government could offer half the fee they pay to private nursing homes to individuals who volunteer to care for a relative, but how such care would be monitored would become an issue.

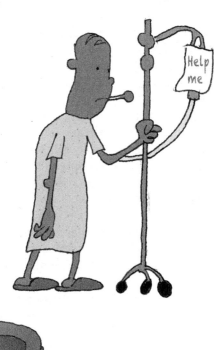

16

Dilemmas of care

Malpractice may also be unintentional, yet based on decisions made with good intentions, by the care assistant or nurse (Dimon 2006). In these situations, the decision of the patient is overridden. This may not legally be done unless allowed under the Mental Care Act, Deprivation of liberty Safeguards, or Mental Health Act, in certain situations, and involving specific procedures. Reasons for overriding patient's wishes may be due to a reluctance to take risks, or an adherence to the medical model of care. Situations may concern patients going out alone, and may involve risk assessments. Issues arise regarding level of mental capacity, which is not easy to determine.

It is possible that some individuals seek power, and actually enjoy mistreating individuals. Burger (1989) suggests that some individuals prefer to control others. Agich (1990) suggests that some nurses are over-protective or paternalistic toward patients, and so will not allow them to make decisions.

Covert practice refers to hiding medication in food or beverages so that it goes undetected by the person receiving the medication. Pills may be crushed or medication in liquid form may be used (Griffith et al 2003). This practice exclusively applies to individuals who are not capable of consenting to treatment. It is intended to ensure that individuals refusing treatment, as a result of their illness, will have access to effective medical treatment. Those who are in favour of this approach argue that it is far less intrusive than administering an injection by physical restraint. The NMC has addressed this issue by producing guidelines (NMC 2012b), to use in conjunction with the Mental Capacity Act (2005), and the NMC code of conduct (2008).

An increase in the use of restraint by nurses may be linked to increased work pressure linked to staff shortages. Dementia patients are increasingly being "restrained" by hospital staff and carers. A report by the CQC revealed that 4,951 "restraining orders" were granted to hospitals and care homes in 2011/2012, up from 3,297 in 2009/10 (Borland 2012).

The orders include locking patients in rooms, fixing seat belt-like devices to chairs, or using powerful sedative drugs to prevent them from wandering. Because the measures technically breach patients' human rights, staff are required by law to get permission from their local authority or NHS trust before taking action. But the CQC warned many patients were being restrained illegally, because hospital and care home staff had not sought approval beforehand. Its inspectors found one distressed woman at a care home in the West Midlands who had been put in a bed with railings so high she could not reach objects from her bedside table.

17

The exploitation of overseas nurses

Nurses from overseas who come to work in British hospitals and care homes face racism, exploitation and isolation, a report claims. Many are also charged large and often illegal fees by recruiters who brought them to the UK, leaving them feeling "manipulated and cheated", says the Royal College of Nursing. Its report – We Need Respect, Experiences of internationally recruited nurses in the UK (2003) – found that many of those questioned describe their employment, both in the NHS and the private sector, as "slavery". Their countries of origin must also be considered because nurses coming here, leaves a shortage there (Shield, Watson 2007).

The report complements previous RCN ones concerning International recruitment: United Kingdom case study (RCN 2002), and Here to stay? International nurses in the UK (RCN 2003). The report explores the motivations and experiences of 67 IRNs, in order to understand why overseas nurses come to work in the UK, what experiences they have, and whether they plan to stay in the UK, return to their countries of origin, or go to another country to work.

Among the problems highlighted is the poor accommodation given to internationally recruited nurses, and a lack of personal support, reinforcing "feelings of isolation and homesickness". The nurses reported experiences of discrimination, sometimes as "crude racism", but also in the way they felt excluded by their British colleagues. They were also singled out for special negative attention if they made any mistakes. The level of support given by the NHS is generally approved of by those questioned, but experiences in the private sector were strongly criticised.

The nurses, though fully qualified in their own countries, with an average of 14 years' experience, were made to undergo an adaptation programme to work in the UK, believing that it would lead to them gaining registration as a nurse. But many who paid thousands of pounds to recruiters to secure adaptation often ended up as low-paid carers in independent care homes, and often reported bullying from other workers, and a feeling of being "policed". Those working in the NHS felt frustrated that they were not allowed to use the nursing skills which they practised in their home countries.

Many said they felt British nurses had poorer working conditions, and longer hours, compared to other places where they had worked. RCN (2003b), based on 10 case studies involving NHS and non NHS managers, identifies the main challenges of managers regarding overseas nurses – language, difference in technical and clinical skills, racism, and reaction to patients. Difference in attitudes may apply to such areas as pain relief and restraint.

Conclusion and further recommendations

It can be stressed again that this author has not approached the subject of poor nursing care through a political bias; whatever detracts from good care should be the concern of all nurses, and, therefore, in this regard, nursing and nurses cannot be apolitical. Many of the recent changes to healthcare provision are the result of neoliberal approaches, and when these prove to adversely affect patient care, as exampled in this book, they should be challenged by nurses, for not to do so is not to promote what is in the best interest of patients. Some measures of privatisation may be in patients' interests, for what matters is good care, wherever that takes place, yet many of the recent reforms seem to have been enacted speedily, and services put out to tender have resulted in private companies operating services on the lowest costs possible.

Some of the following conclusions and recommendations, additional to those suggested in the text, are based on an opposition to changes brought about by political dogma which is leading to an apartheid system of healthcare, with "winners" who can afford private health insurance being segregated from "losers" who cannot. These changes are being introduced on a tide of neoliberal rhetoric which crudely attempts to divide people through targeting the self-interest motive of the young, who "shouldn't have to shoulder the burden of the elderly"; and of the poor working class, who "shouldn't have to support scivers". To divide is to rule. Government announcements through the Department of Health website read like something from Orwell's Ministry of Truth. This is not to oppose neoliberalist doctrine *per se*, and its imperative to privatise; it is to oppose *any doctrine* that makes poor nursing care more likely. There is no reason why private healthcare facilities cannot provide excellent nursing care. Yet, putting all services out to tender is only to invite bids from companies whose financial health is often disguised behind a mountain of debt: the largest care home groups are in debt to the tune of billions; rampant acquisitions of smaller groups of homes has been no more of a success than a comparative situation in the banking industry. Private care facilities need *some* regulation that impacts on their costs, such as imposing minimum levels of staff, and making it compulsory to replace "sick" staff with staff from an "emergency" agency, who can be booked at short notice. The attitude of nurse "let's roll up our sleeves and get on with it" has always been a part of nursing, and sometimes a necessary and good one, but there is evidence of care homes permanently not covering staff shortages; of hospital managers doing the same, and of altering patient dependency levels to cover up *real* staff shortage. Yet, to suggest anything that increases business costs is anathema to the "text book" free marketeer. Theirs is only one vision of privatisation; a less absolute one which recognises that good care can be promoted through *some* regulation effecting costs is another. This author has worked in NHS facilities which gave poor care, and in private facilities that gave good care. It is not a matter of where care takes place, it is a matter of how care is regulated so as to promote good care; not that regulation by itself is a guarantor of good care, for that also depends on the attitude and motivations of those giving care. *Nursing also needs to return to nursing the patient.*

Returning the nurse to patient care. As suggested by Shield and Watson (2007), there is a need to return the role of an enrolled nurse. All nurses should take the enrolled nurse route, during which training their level of compassion, as much as their clinical skills, could be assessed. This author does not take a political stance on this issue. Although disagreeing with the neoliberal influences that are effectively privatising the NHS by stealth, and leading to a "winners" and "losers" healthcare market, the issue facing any government, of any political persuasion, is how to finance the cost of a rapidly expanding elderly population. Nursing followed a route advocated by senior nurses, who sought higher status and rewards for nurses, from which sprang the graduate nurse system. This has become a self-perpetuating monster: An ever-growing number of nurse lecturers support 20,000 nursing students, many of whom will not find employment as a nurse. As mentioned, nursing students on some clinical placements are told to do "management jobs" and not spend time on patient care. During clinical placements, students have academic assignments to complete, and many students also have children to go home to after their clinical shift. This places an intolerable burden of some students. An enrolled nurse trainee would be free to concentrate on what really matters; *good nursing care delivered with a compassionate attitude.* This has always been the goal of nursing, but, sadly, as become too often forgotten.

To those that justify the present nurse graduate system on the grounds that the trainee spends 50% of their time in clinical placements, it can be asked, doing what? And why only 50%? The defence of the current system on the grounds of nursing becoming more "technical", and therefore requires graduates, is hollow; our society has become more "technical", and many young people who do not have a degree could easily master the "technicalities" of nursing, nor would it take them three years to do so. At the end of a two year enrolled nurse programme, those with an academic aptitude, as well as good practical and people skills, could be recommended for a further two year part-time course leading to a degree. They would be guaranteed a post as a nursing sister or charge nurse. All who complete the enrolled nurse programme would be similarly guaranteed a job. They would have the necessary hands-on experience to "hit the ground running", and not be discriminated against in applying for their first job, which is what the present situation allows. Enrolled nurse training could be locally based, with schools of nursing being linked to their local NHS hospital, in which students would be fully counted as staff in their clinical placements, and would supplement, not replace, care assistants, thus increasing staff/patient ratios. One week in "school" followed by two months of ward work would be a practical ratio of training; with, perhaps, three academic projects to be completed over a two year period, to be assessed at diploma level. "Technical" practice would be gained, as an example, by taking blood pressures of poorly patients, and not "dummies", or fellow (healthy) students.

Such a return to an older system of training would have to be countered by safeguards that the old system lacked. Too often the old schools of nursing would be staffed by lecturers who had trained with those in charge of hospital wards where students undertook placements, and this closeness could lead to students' complaints about poor care on wards being dismissed. The complaints procedure in schools of nursing would have to be subject to the scrutiny of an independent, local organisation, such as Healthwatch. The marking of assignments would similarly be subject to independent scrutiny; a percentage of them are currently externally marked.

The selection procedure to enter nursing would place emphasis on the importance of compassionate care, and thorough questioning of an entrants' motives would be undertaken. Pay would be a little better than commensurate with a diploma level job, so as to recognise the value given to care by society. Nurses would be respected by giving *good nursing care delivered with a compassionate attitude*. The old system of nurse training had many faults, many documented within this book, but what it required was a radical reform to place checks on "institutional" and impersonal care; not a replacement by a costly system that was too much about increasing the prestige of those who advocated it.

The government suggest it neither adequately protects its members as a trade union, nor protects vulnerable patients: "Consider the Royal College of Nursing's foot-stamping response to the Health Secretary's plan for all trainee nurses to spend 12 months working as a healthcare assistant, to teach them the fundamental importance of ensuring patients are washed and comfortable. It is so obsessed with nursing being treated as an academic pursuit that it risks giving the damaging impression that performing simple acts of kindness, like feeding and cleaning patients, is now beneath its members. Of course, nurses should be properly trained, and rewarded, for their work. But, if the RCN really believes that paper qualifications are more valuable to patients than human compassion, it has forgotten why the NHS was founded in the first place" (dailymail.co.uk 2013).

Nurses and care staff are dispensable: "It had come to his knowledge, he said, that a foolish and wicked rumour had been circulated at the time of Boxer's removal. Some of the animals had noticed that the van which took Boxer away was marked "Horse Slaughterer," and had actually jumped to the conclusion that Boxer was being sent to the knacker's. It was almost unbelievable, said Squealer, that any animal could be so stupid. Surely, he cried indignantly, whisking his tail and skipping from side to side, surely they knew their beloved Leader, Comrade Napoleon, better than that? But the explanation was really very simple. The van had previously been the property of the knacker, and had been bought by the veterinary surgeon, who had not yet painted the old name out. That was how the mistake had arisen" (Orwell 1951).

References

Aei.gov.au. National Office of Overseas Skills Recognition. Australian Government. Web: aei.gov.au/services-and-resources 22 April 2013. (From Anne Melano via Linkedin 2013).

Age UK (2013). Hospital Discharge Arrangements. Factsheet 37. Web: ageuk.org.uk. February 2013.

Agich, G. J. C. (1993). Autonomy in Longterm Care USA. Oxford University Press.

Aha.org (2011). Fast Facts On US Hospitals. Web: aha.org/research 1 April 2013.

Ahern, K. McDonald, S . (2002). The Beliefs of Nurses Who Were Involved in a Whistleblowing Event. Journal of Advanced Nursing 38 (3) pp. 303–309.

Aihw.org Web: aihw.org/haag09–10/numberofhospitals. 11 February 2013.

Allnurses.com (2012). Lazy Stuck Up Nurses. 9 February 2012.

Alzheimers.org.uk. Web: alzheimers.org.uk. 14 April 2013.

Alzheimers.org.uk. Human Rights Issues Arising From The Treatment of Old Persons in Hospital and Residential Care. Web: alzheimers.org.uk. 4 April 2013.

Aoa.gov.uk (2012). Long-term Care Ombudsman Programme. 2 March 2013.

Asch, S. E. (1951). Effects of group pressure on the modification and distortion of judgments. In H. Guetzkow (Ed.), Groups, leadership and men (pp. 177–190). Pittsburgh, PA: Carnegie Press.

Australian Government Department of Health and Ageing (2002). Ageing In Place Quality Care for Older Australians. Web: health.gov.au. 2 March 2013.

Bartek, J. K. Linderman, M. Newton, M. Fitzgerald, A. P. Hawks, J. H. (1988) Nurse-Identified Problems in the Management of Alcoholic Patients, Journal of Studies on Alcohol v. 49 n. 1 pp. 63–70.

Bayne Powell, R .(1951). Travellers in 18th Century England. London. J Murray.

bbc.co.uk (2013). Private Ambulances 'Risk Patient Safety' Web: 21 April 2013.

BBC news (2010). Customers Losing Thousands on Pensions Fees, Commissions. Web: bbc.co.uk. 4 October 2012.

BBC news (2011). RCN: NHS Care Assistants 'Training Unacceptable'. Web: bbc.co.uk. 2 April 2013.

BBC news (2013). Private Ambulances 'Risk Patient Safety'. Web: bbc.co.uk. 2 May 2013.

Bennet, C. (1980). Nursing Home Life: What it is and What it could be. New York. Tiresias Press.

Beresford, P. (2011). From 'No Such Thing As Society' To 'Big Society': Spot The Difference. Web: guardian.co.uk. 2 March 2013.

Berry, Rev. J. C. (2012). Care of The Vulnerable Elderly. The Crisis In Modern Medicine. Catholic Medical Quarterly v. 62, n. 1. February 2012.

big-lies.org/UK-private-hospitals (nd) Private Hospitals In Britain 2 May 2013.

Bloxham, A. (2011). Man With Down's Syndrome Ignored After He Was Detained in Hospital and locked Up Before He Died. The Telegraph 23 November 2012.

bmartin (nd) Nurses In The Aged Care System. Web: bmartin.cc/dissent.1 February 2013.

Boehm, D. A. (2008). The safety net of the safety net: How federally qualified health centers "subsidize" Medicaid managed care. Medical Anthropology Quarterly, 19 (1), pp. 47–63.

Boffey, D. (2013) NHS Hospitals In Bid To treat Far More NHS Patients. The Guardian 6 April 2012.

Bokhari (nd). A Comparative Study of Ombudsman Office in Australia, Pakistan and UK. Web: policy.hu/bkhari/project. 23 June 2012.

Bond, S. Bond, J. (1996). Outcomes of Care Within a Multiple Care Study in the Evaluation of the Experimental NHS Nursing Home. Age and Aging v. 19 pp. 11–18.

Borland, S. (2011). Elderly Facing Eviction From NHS Beds. Web: dailymail.co.uk/health/NHS-evict elderly blocking hospital beds.16 February 2011.

Borland, S. (2012). Locked up and Sedated; Huge Rise in Number of Dementia Patients Being 'Restrained' By Hospital Staff and Carers. Web: dailymail.co/dementia-care. 24 March 2012.

Bosely, S. (2012). NHS: Forgetting Needs of Care Home Residents, Warns Review. The Guardian 7 March 2012.

Boyle, G. (2010). Social Policy For People With Dementia In England Promoting Human Rights? Health and Social Care in The Community 18 (5) pp. 511–519.

Brodaty, H. Draper, B. Low, L. F. (2003). Nursing home staff attitudes towards residents with dementia: strain and satisfaction with work, J. Adv. Nurs. December 2003; 44 (6) pp. 583–90.

Brooke, V. (1989). How Elders Adjust: Through What Phases Do Newly Admitted Residents Pass? Geriatric Nursing (10) pp. 66–68.

Buckland, L . (2012). Foreign Nurses Soar By 40% as NHS is Hit By Shortage of Trained Staff. Web: mailonline 9 January 2009.

Burger, J. M. (1989). Negative Reactions to Increases in Perceived Control. Journal of Personal and Social Psychology v. 56 n. 2 pp. 246–256.

Calkin, S. (2013). Local Healthwatch 'Bound and Gagged'. Health Service Journal 11 January 2013.

Callaghan, M. (2003). Nursing Morale: What is it Like and Why? Journal of Advanced Nursing 42 (1) pp. 82–89.

Campbell, D. (2013a). Hospitals Must Shrink or Shut. The Guardian 8 April 2013.

Campbell, D. (2013). Nurses Must spend a Year on Basic Care. The Guardian 26 March 2013.

Carter, P. (2013). Overworked NHS Nurses Not To Blame For Mid Staffs Scandal. The Guardian 6 February 2013.

Carvel, J. (2012). Stafford Hospital Investigator Berates CQC Regulator. Web: gaurdian.co.uk/news. 22 July 2012.

Chandra, N. (2012) Nurse Enrollment Under Scanner Over Fake OBC Certificates.

Web: Indiatoday.intoday.in/india. 28 July 2012.

Chapman, J. C. (2013). Victory For NHS Whistlelowers: After Daily Mail Campaign Health Secretary Bans Gagging Orders on NHS Staff. Daily Mail 13 March 2013

Cheek, J. Ballantyne, A. Jones, J. Roder-Allen, G. Kitto, S. (2013). Ensuring Excellence: An Investigation Of The Issues That Impact On The Registered Nurse Providing Residential Care To Older Australians. International Journal of Nursing Practice (2) pp. 103–111.

CHRE report (2012). Strategic Review of the Nursing and Midwifery Council Final Report 3 July 2012.

Chubb, E. (2009) Nursing Without Caring. Web: compassionincare.com/news 3 September 2009.

Clarke, T. Kellaher, M. Fairbrother, G. (2010). Starting a Care Improvement Journey; Focusing on The Essentials Of Bedside Nursing Care in an Australian Teaching Hospital. Journal of Clinical Nursing 19 July 2010.

Cliffirdbeersfoundation.co.uk. Web: 1 April 2013.

Clough, R. (1981). Old Age Homes London. George Allen and Unwin.

Collins, N. (2012). NHS Patients Get 'Unacceptable' Care From Care Assistants. The Telegraph 5 November 2011.

Complaintline.com.au Health services complaints. Web: 1 May 2013.

Connelly, K. (2012). Germany "Export" Old and Sick To Foreign Care Homes. Web: guardian.co.uk. 22 March 2013.

Cornwell, J. (2012). The King's Fund. Web: Kingsfund.org.uk. 1 May 2013.

Considine, M. (2001). Enterprising states: The public management of Welfare-to-Work. Cambridge: Cambridge University Press.

Cotton, C. in Morgan, J. (2011). How Well Are Our Police Officers Paid? Web: bbcnews.co.uk. 8 March 2011.

Coughlin, T. A., Zuckeman, S. (2008). State responses to new flexibility in Medicaid. The Millbank Quarterly, 86 (2), pp. 209–240.

CQC (nd). Our Action Since Winterbourne View. Web: cqc.org.uk. 22 April 2013.

CQC (2010). 34 care homes and eight care agencies shut down ahead of tough new registration system, says Care Quality Commission. Web: cqc.org.uk 22 April 2013.

CQC (2011). How to Complain about a Health or Social Care Service. Web: cqc.org.uk. 22 April 2013.

CQC (2012). Annual Report and Accounts 2011/2012. Web: cqc.org 14 March 2013.

CQC (2013). Healthwatch. Web: cqcorg.uk. 1 April 2013.

Currentnursing.com (2012). Development of Nursing Theories (includes Lancaster and Lancaster 1981) Web: currentnursing.com/nursing 14 February 2012.

Currie, L. Watts, C. (2012) Preceptorship and Pre-Registration Nursing Education. Web: Williscommission.org.uk. 2 May 2013.

Curzio, J. Baillie, L. (2009). A Survey Of First Year Student Nurses' Experiences Of Learning Blood Pressure Measurement. Nurse Education in Practice (9) pp. 61–71.

Dailymail.co.uk (2013). Nursing Union That Puts Patient Care Last. Web: dailymail.co.uk. 22 April 2013.

Dean, E. (2012). Regular Ward Checks Raise Standards Of Care. Nursing Management v. 19 n. 2 pp. 12–16.

De Bellis, A. (2010). Australian Residential Aged Care And The Quality of Nursing Care Provision. Contemporary Nurse v. 35 Issue 1 pp.100–113.

De Bellis, A. (2006). Behind Open Doors: A Construct of Nursing Practice in an Australian Residential Aged Care Facility. Unpublished PHD theses Flinders University, Adelaide, Australia. Includes Ronalds (1989).

DeForge, R. Van Wyk, P. Hall, J. Salmoni, A . (2011). Afraid To Care: Unable to Care: A Critical Ethnography Within A Long-Term Care Home. Journal of Aging Studies (25) pp. 515–426.

De La Cuesta, C. (1983). The Nursing Process From Development To Implementation. Journal of Advanced Nursing September (8) pp. 365–371.

Department of Health (2001). Care Homes for Older People. National Minimum Standards. Care Standards Act 2000. London. The Stationary Office.

Department of Health (2010). Preceptorship Framework For Newly Qualified Nurses, Midwives and Allied Health Professionals. London. The Stationary Office.

Department of Health (2010). Essence of Care. Web: dh.gov.uk 1 March 2013.

Department of Health (2013a). Charities Join Forces in Push for Greater People Power in Local Health and Care Services. Web: Healthandcare.dh.gov.uk. 4 April 2013.

Department of Health (2013b). Press release: Putting Patients First: government publishes response to Francis Report. 3 April 2013.

Diamond, T. (1992). Making Grey Gold. The University of Chicago Press.

Dimon, C. (2005). The Challenging Role of The Care Home Manager. Nursing and Residential Care December. v. 7 n. 12 p. 571.

Dimon, C. (2006). Decisions and Dilemmas in Care Homes. Oxford. Fivepin.

Dimond, B. (2005). Exploring Common Deficiencies That Occur in Record Keeping. British Journal of Nursing pp. 568–570.

Donnelly, L. Leach, B. (2013). English Test Course Could See EU Doctors Barred From Britain. Web: telegraph.co.uk. 1 March 2013.

Donnelly, L. Moore, A. (2013). Hospital Pays £1800 A Day For A Nurse In NHS Staff Crisis. The Telegraph. 19 January 2013.

Dowbiggin, I. R .(2011). In Defence of Institutions. Web: Psychologytoday.com 11 December 2011.

Dubree, M. Vogelpohl, R. (1980). When Hope Dies — So Might The Patient. Am. J. Nurs. November. 80 (11) pp. 2046–9.

ECCA. Web: ecca.org.uk. (2012). Local Healthwatch (LHW) Regulations Press release. 9 October 2012.

Economicsabout.com (nd). The Decline of Union Power. Web: 13 March 2013.

Edenalternative. Web: edenalternative.co.uk. 1 February 2013.

Ed24.co.uk (2013) pensions. 8 March 2013.

Emirates24/7.com. Fraud: 56 Fake Doctors, Nurses Caught in Dubai. Web: euro.who.int. 4 December 2011.

England.nhs.uk. How to make a complaint to NHS England. Web: England.nhs.uk/contact-us/complaint. 20 March 2013.

Equality and Human Rights Commission Close to Home: An Inquiry into Old people and Human Rights in Home Care: An executive Summary. Web: equalityhumanrights.com 20 March 2013.

Fleming, G. (2009). Nurses Need Degrees, Like a Hole in the Head. Web: Nursing Times.net. 20 September 2009.

Ford, S. (2011). Whistleblowing nurse Wins £15,000 Payout After Unfair Dismissal. Web: nursingtimes.net. 6 October 2011.

Ford, S. (2013a). Exclusive: student opinion divided over need to work as HCA. Web: NursingTimes.net. 17 April 2013.

Ford, S. (2013b). Full Survey Results: Are You Safe To Speak Out? Web: nursingtimes.net/whistleblower 12 March 2013.

Ford, S. (2013c). RCN 'Acutely Aware' of Lessons From Francis Report. Web: nursingtimes.net/hone/francis-report. 6 February 2013.

Ford Rojas, J. P. (2011). Residents at short-staffed care homes 'woken at 4am'. Web: telegraph.co.uk. 11 December 2011.

Formato, P. (2002). The Step Up in Enforcement of Nursing Homes Recent Survey Trends. Web: abramslaw.com/CM/Articles 3 June 2012.

Foundation For Quality Care (2013). Nursing Home Artists Honoured in 2013 Annual Calendar. Web: theffqc.org. 4 January 2013.

Francis, R. (2013). Public Inquiry Report of the Mid Staffordshire NHS Foundation Trust Public Inquiry. Exec Summary v. 1. The Stationary Office 6 February 2013.

Gaffney, D. (2012). Benefits Spending: a Quick History. Web: Stumblingandmumblingtypepad.com 1 January 2012.

Glasper, E .A. (nd). Regulating Health Care Support Workers: Is the Government Listening. Web: soton.academia.edu. 16 August 2012.

Goffman, E. (1961). Asylums. Penguin USA.

Graham, J. M. (1983). Experimental Nursing Homes for Elderly people in the NHS. Age and Ageing v. 12 pp. 273–274.

Grey, M. (2011). The changing face of social welfare and social work in Australia. ERIS web journal. The University of Newcastle, New South Wales, Australia.

Griffin, A. (2007). UK Nears European Average in Proportion of GDP Spent on Health Care. BMJ 334 (7591) 442.

Griffith, R. Griffiths, H. Jordan, S. (2003) Administration of medicines part 1: the law and nursing. Nursing Standard v. 18 n. 2 pp. 47–53.

Griffiths, P. Robinson, S. (2010). Moving Forward With Health Care Support and Workforce Regulation.

Grimes, R. (2013). Why is the government preparing for a dramatic rise in NHS patients going private. Web: Opendemocracy.net 22 April 2013.

Gubrium, J. F.(1975). Living and Dying at Murray Manor. St Martins Press. New York.

hadsco.wa.gov.au Health and Disability Services Complaints Office. 22 March 2013.

Hardy, L. K. (1986). Identifying The Place of Theoretical Frameworks in an Evolving Discipline. Journal of Advanced Nursing January v. 11 n. 1. pp. 103–107.

Harrington, C. (2001). Residential Nursing Facilities in The US. BMJ September 323 (7311) pp. 507–510.

Harrison, A. (2013). Warning of rise of Unqualified Teachers in Classrooms. Web: bbcnews.co.uk. 31 March 2013.

Hart, C. (2013). Twenty Years On, It's Time We Stopped Asking in Unison. Web: nursingtimes.net/Chris-hart 12 March 2013.

Havig, A. K. Skogsgad, A. K. Jekshu, L. E. Romoren, T. I. (2011). Leadership, staffing and quality of care in nursing homes. BMC Health Services Research 2011 11 (327). Web: Biomedcentral.com. 22 February 2013.

Hennessy, P. Donnelly, L. (2013). Seventeen NHS Hospitals Have Dangerously low Levels of Nurses. Web: telegraph.co.uk. 12 January 2013.

Heine, C. A. (1986). Burnout Among Nursing Home Personnel. Journal of Gerontological Nursing 12 (93) pp. 14–18.

Hiranandani, V. S. (2011). Disabling healthcare? Medicaid managed care and people with disabilities in America. Poverty & Public Policy, 3 (2) article 7.

Hitchcock, T. Howard, S. Shoemaker, R. (2012). Parish Nurses. Londonlives 1690–1800. Web: londonlives.org. 17 June 2012.

Holahan, J. (2009). Medicaid and entitlement reform. The Health Policy Center. The Urban Institute.

Horton, E .S. (2007). Neoliberalism And The Australian Healthcare System. Conference of The Philosophy of Education Society of Australasia, Wellington, New Zealand. Web: eprints.qut.edu.au.12 February 2013.

Howard, J. Strauss, A. (eds) (1975). Humanising Health Care. New York. J Wiley and Sons.

Hung, R. (nd) Caring About Strangers: A Lingisan Reading of Kaffka's Metamorphosis. University of Hawaii Web: 2.hawaii.edu.peaconf 12 February 2013.

Hunter, R. (2012). Neglect and Abuse in Aged Care. The Drum Opinion. Web: abc.net.au/unleashed 3 February 2012.

Imison, C. Ashton, B. Steward, K. Willis, A. (2011). Good Governance For Clinical Commissioning Groups An Introductory Guide. London. The King's Fund.

Isaacs, S. R. Jellinek, P. (2007). Is There a (Volunteer) Dr in the House? Free Clinics and Volunteer Physician Referral Networks in the US. Health Affairs v. 27 n. 3 pp. 871–876. Web: content.health-affairs.org.

Jackson, D. Peters, K. Andrew, S. Edenborough, M. Halcomb, E. Luck, L.. Salamanson, Y. Wilkes, L. (2010). Understanding Whistleblowing: Qualitative Insights From Nurse Whistleblowers 2194–2201 (66) (10).

Jewkes, R. Abrahams, N. Mvo, Z. (1998). Why Do Nurses Abuse Patients? Reflections From South African Obstetric Services. Soc. Sci. Med. v. 47 n. 11 pp. 1781–1795. Web: tractionproject.org. 17 February 2013.

Journal of Anaesthesia practice (2011). News: Protecting the NHS for future generations – services only for the poor are poor services. Web: japractice.co.uk April 2011.

Kada, S. Nygaard, H. A. Mukesh, B. N. Geituing, J. T. (2009). Staff Attitudes Towards Institutionalised Dementia Residents. Journal of Clinical Nursing 18.8 (16) pp. 2383–92.

Kaffka, F. (1972). Metamorphosis. Bantam Classics.

Kawam, E. (2012). The Rise of Neoliberal Rhetoric and the Intersection of Modern Day Medicaid Priority: A Study of Young Residents in Nursing Homes. Disability Studies Quarterly v 32 n. 1.

Kim, H. Marcus, H. R. (1999). Deviance or Uniqueness, Harmony or Conformity? A Cultural Analysis. Journal of Personality and Social Psychology. 77 (4) pp. 785–800.

King, I .M. (1971). Towards a Theory for Nursing USA. J Wiley and Sons.

King, K. The Golden Experience. Web: thegoldenexperience. 1 February 2013.

Kosciejew, R. J. (2012). The Designing Theory of Transference v. 11 p. 132. Web:scribd.com. 1 March 2013.

Krause, M. R. Palmer, J. L. Bowers, B. J. Buckwalter, K. C. (2011). Responding to Poor-Quality Care During Research In Nursing homes. Research in Gerontological Nursing v. 4 Issue 1 pp. 47–52.

Laird, C. (1982). Limbo.California. Chandler and Sharp.

Laurance, J. (2012). Private hospital told doctors to delay NHS work to boost profits The Independent 21 July 2012.

Lee-Treweek, G. (1992). Bedroom Abuse: The Hidden Work in a Nursing Home. Generations Review pt. 2 v. 4 pp. 2–4.

Levett- Jones, T. Lathlean, J. (2009). 'Don't Rock the Boat': Nursing Students' Experiences of Conformity and Compliance. Nurse Education Today (29) 342–349.

Lievesley, N. Crosby, G. Bowman, C . (2011). The Changing Roles of Care Homes BUPA and CPA. Web: cpa.org.uk/information/reviews 1 March 2013.

Littlejohn, C. (2012). Are Nursing models To Blame For Low Morale? Nursing Standard v. 16 n. 17 pp. 39–41.

Lin, J. (2010). Honor or Abandon: Societies' Treatment of Elderly Intrigues Scholar. UCLA Today (1.7)

Local Government Ombudsman. Web: lgo.org.uk. 1 March 2013.

Local Government Ombudsman (2012). An Analysis Of Complaints Statistics 2011/2012. Web: ltombudsman.org.uk. 1 March 2013.

Lucero, R. J. Lake, E. T. & Aiken, L.H. (2009). Variations in nursing care quality across hospitals. Journal of Advanced Nursing. 65 (11): 2299–310.

Lythe, R. (2013). Thousands Of Care Home Residents Told to Pay More or Move Out Because of The Squeeze on Council Budgets. Web: mailonline. 1 March 2013.

MacDonald, S. Ahern, K. (2000). The Professional Consequences of Whistleblowing By Nurses. J. Prof. Nurse Nov-Dec 16 (6) pp. 312–21.

MacDonald, V. (2011). Leaked Document Shows How Doctors Can Profit From NHS Reform. Web: channel4.com. 2 March 2013.

Mandelstam, M. (2012). How We Treat The Sick: Neglect and Abuse in our Health Services. Jessica Kingsley

Martin, D. (2009). All New Nurses Will Need To Have Degrees To Work For The NHS (But Will It Benefit Patients?). Web: dailymail.co.uk/news. 13 November 2009.

Martin, D. (2011). Language Test For All Foreign Drs: Law Will Bar Medics Who Can't Speak English. Web: dailymail.co.uk. 1 March 2013.

Martin, J. P. (1984). Hospitals in Trouble. Basil Blackwell.

Mason, R. (2013). Mid Staffs: Labour Government ignored MP requests for public inquiry into deaths. The Telegraph 17 February 2013.

Maslach, C. Santee, R. T. Wade, C. (1987). Individuation, Gender Role, and Dissent. Psychology 53 (6) pp. 1088–1093.

Matthews, J. C. (2009). UK v USA -The Basic Healthcare Facts. Web: liberalconspiracy.org. 14 August 2009.

McCance, T. McCormack, B. Dewing, J. (2011). An Exploration of Person-Centredness In Practice. Online Journal Of Issues In Nursing v. 16 n. 2. Web:nursingworld.org. 1 March 2013.

McFarlane, J. (2013). Freeze on foreign nurses as NHS chiefs admit they have no idea how many lied about qualifications and experience using fake IDs. Web: mailonline 10 March 2013.

McGregor, K . (2011). Up to 200,000 Care Assistants Paid Below Minimum Rate. Community Care 3 October 2011.

Meikle, J. (2011). Foreign Nurses Registering in UK Despite a 20 year work Gap. Web: guardian.co.uk. 2 September 2011.

Menzies, I. E. P. (1970). The Functioning of Social Systems as a Defence Against Anxiety, Tavistock.

Middleton, J. (2012). 'The Regulator Must Not Be Seen as an HR Service'. Web: nursingtimes.net/opinion 2 March 2013.

Milne, S. (2012). The problem with unions is They're Not Strong Enough. The Guardian 11 September 2012.

Miskin, P. (2013). Enriching Clinical Nursing Education through Simulation. Web: nursetogether.com. 3 March 2013.

Morgan, J. (2011). How Well Are Our Police Officers Paid? Web: bbcnews.co.uk. 8 March 2011. Includes Cotton, C.

Morris, H. O. (nd) Nurses Unions As an Indirect Predictor of Patient Satisfaction: A Nurse's Perspective. Web: nursestogether.com. 1 March 2013.

Morris, P. (1969). Put Away – A Sociological Study Of Institutions Of The Mentally Retarded. London, Routledge and Kegan Paul.

Mums.net. Web: mums.net. 15 March 2013.

Naish, J. (2012a). Rogue Nurses Who Attack and Steal From Patients Handed 'License To Abuse' As Report Reveals How Few Are Actually Struck Off. Web: dailymail.co.uk. 22 February 2013.

Naish, J. (2012b). The doctor and nurses putting lives at risk because they can't speak English. Web: mailonline. 31 March 2012.

Nationmaster.com. Web: nationmaster.com. 1 February 2013.

Newton, G. (1979). This Bed My Centre. Virago.

NHS for sale (2013). What's The Impact? Web: nhsforsale.info.

Nichols, K. (1992). Understanding Support. Nursing Times. March 25. v. 88 n. 13 pp. 34–35.

NMC (2006). Circular: NMC Recommends Preceptorship. Web: nmc.uk.org. 1 May 2013.

NMC (2008). Standards To Support Learning and Assessment In Practice. Web: nmc.uk.org. 1 May 2013.

NMC (2010a). Standards For Pre-Registration Nursing Education. Web: nmc.uk.org. 1 May 2013.

NMC (2010b). Essential Skills Clusters Web: nmc.uk.org.1 May 2013

NMC (2008). The Code Standards Of Conduct, Performance and Ethics For Nurses and midwives. London. NMC.

NMC (2012a). Annual Fitness To Practice Report 2011–2012. London. TSO.

NMC (2012b). Covert Administration of Medicines. Web: nmc.uk.org. 1 May 2013.

NMC (2013a). Trained Outside Europe. Web: nmc.uk.org/registration. 4 April 2013.

NMC (2013b). Update; Overseas Registration of Nurses and midwives Web: nmc-uk.org. 1 March 2013.

NMC (2013c). Adaptation and Aptitude Test. Web: nmc.uk.org. 22 March 2013.

NMC (2013). NMC Resumes Overseas Application Processes. 9 April 2013.

Noddings, N. (1984). Caring: A Feminine Approach To Ethics And Moral Education. University of California Press.

Norbergh, K. G. Helin, Y. Dahl, A. Hellzén, O. Asplund, K . (2006). Nurses' attitudes towards people with dementia: the semantic differential technique. Nurse Ethics. May; 13 (3) pp. 264–74.

Nursing In Practice (2012). NMC Withdraws Telephone and Advisory Service. 22 June 2012.

Nursing Standard (2013). Challenges of Bad Practice. Web: nursingstandard.rcnpublishing.co.uk. 1 March 2013.

O'Connor, S. (2011). Human Cost Forgotten in Race To Invest. Web: ft.com. 30 May 2011.

Odone, C. (2013). Another NHS scandal: managers rake in a fortune while nurses earn less than the average wage. Web: telegraph.co.uk. 22 April 2013.

OECD (2011). Health at A Glance. Web: Oecd.org. 1 February 2013.

Ombudsman (2011). Care and Compassion. London. Parliamentary and Healthcare Service Ombudsman.

Ombudsman (2012). Listening and Learning: The Ombudsman's Review Of Complaints Handling By The NHS in England 2011–2012. Web: ombudsman.org.uk. 1 March 2013.

Ombudsman (2012b). NHS Fails To Communicate Effectively With Patients and Families, Warns Ombudsman. Web: ombudsman.org.uk. 9 November 2011.

O'Murchu, C. (2011). Neglect Amid Tight Care Home Margins. Web: ft.com/companies. 30 May 2011.

Orwell, G. (1951). Animal Farm. Penguin.

Parliament (2011). The NHS Complaints System is Not Working, Says Commons Health Committee. Web: parliament.uk/a-z/health. 28 June 2011.

Parihar, R. (2012). Degrees of Guilt. India Today. Web: indiatoday.intoday.com. 11 February 2013.

Payley, A. (2012). Elder and Nursing Home Abuse: A Universal Problem. Web: thescavenger.net. 13 March 2012.

Pearl, J. (2011). Care Homes are Failing But is it Hard To Complain? Web: conversation.which.co.uk. 12 January 2013.

Pearson, A. (1992). Nursing at Burford. A Story of Change. Middlesex. Scutari Press.

Peplau, H. E. (1991). Interpersonal Relations in Nursing. Springer. New York.

Perez, P. (2011). Nursing Profession And The Ethics Of Care. Practical Ethics. University of Oxford. Web: blog.practicalethics.ox.ac.uk. 21 February 2011.

Pettinger, T. (2013). The Growth of Welfare Spending in The UK. Web: economicshelp.org.

Phio.org. Web: phio.org.au. 2 February 2013.

Pickover, E. (2012). NHS receives 3000 patient complaints a week. Web: theindependent.co.uk. 28 September 2012.

Popenici, S. Kerr, S. (2013). What Undermines Higher Education And How This Impacts Employment, Economies and our Democracies. Amazon.

Portsmouth.co.uk. (2012). Plans For Wards Rounds By Nurses Welcomed. 1 July 2012.

Price Fishback (2010). Who Spends More on Social Welfare: the United States or Sweden? Web: anthrocivitas.net 26 May 2010.

Prielipp, R. C. Magro, M. Morell, R. C. Brull, S. J. (2010). The Normalization of Deviance: Do We (Un)Knowingly Accept Doing The Wrong Thing? IAANA Journal. August v. 78 n. 4 pp.1499–1502.

Ramesh, R. (2012). NHS Trusts Are Enmeshed In private provision – As Buyers and Suppliers. The Guardian 18 December 2012.

RCN (2003). "We Need Respect": Experiences of Internationally Recruited Nurses In The UK. Web: rcn.org/publications. 1 March 2013.

RCN (2003b). Here To Stay? International Nurses in The UK. Web: rcn.org/publications. 1 March 2013.

RCN (2013). Student Nurses Maintained But Worrying Shortage of Nurses, Warns RCN. Web: rcn.org.uk. 1 March 2013.

REUTERS (2013). RBS to Sell Up to $3 Billion Stake in Citizens Bank. Web: cnbc.com. 1 April 2013.

Richards, E .A.(2011). Stop The Silence Of Elder Abuse. American Nurse Today August v. 6 n. 8.

Robb, B. (1967). Sans Everything. London. AEGIS.

Robb, E. Maxwell, E. Elcock, K. S. (2011). How Skill Mix Affects Quality OF Care. Web: nursingtimes.net. 25 November 2011.

Robinson Wolf, Z. Hughes R. D. (nd) .Chapter 35: Error Reporting and Disclosure. Web: ahrq.gov/professionals. 1 May 2013.

Rogers, S. (2013). UK Welfare Spending: How Much Does Each Benefit Really Cost? The Guardian 8 January 2013.

Ronalds, C. (1989). Residents Rights in Nursing Homes and Hostels Final Report. Canberra. Australian Govt Publishing Service. Reference obtained from De Bellis, A.

Rose, M. E. (1971). The English Poor Law 1780–1936. London. David and Charles.

Ross, T. (2013). 'Hospital Hotels' for 30,000 Elderly Patients. The Telegraph 22 April 2013.

Royal College of Psychiatrists (2008). Study Reveals Cultural Differences in Attitudes Towards Caring For People With Dementia. King's College London. Web: kcl.ac.uk/op/news. 2 September 2008.

Schlesinger, F. (2010). The Nurse Victimised For Being A Whistleblower: Trainee Thrown Out After Exposing Abuse At Shamed Hospital. Web: dailymail.co.uk.15 May 2010.

Scott, H. (2010). The Medical Model: The Right Approach To Service Provision? Mental Health Practice February. v. 13 n. 5 pp. 27–30.

Scullion, P. A. (2009). Models of Disability: Their Influence in Nursing and potential Role in Challenging Discrimination. Ph.D. thesis. Coventry University.

Seekhalakshmi, S. Soshargiri, M. (2006). Fake Nursing Colleges. Web:airmiles.time-sofindia.indiatimes.com. 24 April 2006.

Seligman, M. E. P. (1975). Helplessness: On Depression, Development and Death. San Francisco. W.H. Freeman.

Shah, P. Mountain, D. (2007). The Medical model Is Dead – Long Live The Medical Model. The British Journal of Psychiatry (191) pp. 375–377.

Sharma, S. L. (1989). Perimeter of the Medical Model. Web: szasz.com/sharma 13 June 2012.

Shields, L. Watson, R. (2007). The Demise of Nursing Within The UK: A Warning For Medicine. Journal of Royal Society of Medicine 100 (02) February. pp. 70–74.

Web: ncbi.nlm.nih.gov. J. R. Soc. Med. (122) February 2013.

Shi, L. Singh, D. A. (2003). Delivering Health Care in America: A Systems Approach. 2nd ed. Massachussetts. Jones and Bartlett Publishers.

Shimizutani, M. Odagiri, Y. Ohya, Y. Schimomitsu, T. Kristensen, T. S. Maruta, T. Iimori, M. (2008). Relationship of Nurse Burnout With Personality Characteristics and Coping Behaviours. Industrial Health (46) pp. 326–335.

Sigman, S. J. (2009). Adjustment to the Nursing Home as a Social Interactional Accomplishment. Journal of Applied Communication Research v. 14 issue 1 pp. 37–58.

Smith, P. B. Bond, M. H. (1993). Social Psychology Across Cultures: Analysis and Perspectives. Hemel Hempstead. Harvester Wheatsheaf.

Smith, R. (2011). 5 million Elderly people Only Have TV For Company. The Telegraph 22 November 2011.

Smith, R. (2012a). Nurses lack Compassion NHS Admits. The Telegraph 18 January 2012.

Smith, R. (2012b). Patients 'Put at Risk' By failure Of Nurses Regulator. The Telegraph 3 July 2012.

Squires, R. (2010). Unfed And unwashed; 'Nursing Home Residents Living In Hell'. The Sunday Telegraph. Web: news.com.au. 30 May 2010.

Steffensmeier, D. Allan, E. (1996). Gender and Crime:Toward a Gendered Theory of Female Offending. Ann. Rev. Social. (22) pp. 459–87.

Sweden.SE (nd). Elderly Care: A Challenge For Our Future. Web: sweden.se/eng/home/society/elderly-care. 1 February 2013.

Syal, R. (2011). MPs Fear Return of Southern Cross Home Scandal. The Guardian 6 December 2012.

Taylor, A. (2008). Separation of Residents Still Occurs. Community Care (26) June pp. 25–26.

Taylor, H. (2012). Overseas Nurses Face a Trial of Exploitation and Deportation Despite the Fact NHS is Crying Out For Highly-Trained Healthcare Workers. Overseas Aid. Web: unison.org.uk. 22 January 2013.

The Telegraph (2010). Foreign Nurses To Be Allowed To Work in Britain 'Without Safety Checks' 12 July 2010.

The Patients Association (2009). Patients Not Numbers, People Not Statistics.

Thompson, I. E. Melia, K. Boyd, K. M. (2006). 5th. ed. Nursing Ethics. Edinburgh. Churchill Livingstone.

Timoney, D. (2013). Web: blogspot.co.uk. 17 February 2013.

Topping, A. (2013). Nurses to Make Hourly Rounds Under Cameron Plans. The Guardian 6 January 2013.

Townsend, P. (1962). The Last Refuge. London. Routledge and Kegan Paul.

Triggle, N. (2011). Basic Home Care Help 'Breaching Human Rights'. Web: bbc.co.uk. 23 November 2011.

Triggle, N. (2012). Quality of Care Suffering says Regulator. Web: bbc.co.uk. 23 November 2011.

Triggle, N. (2013). Healthcare Assistants 'Want Professional Register'. Web: bbcnews. 11 April 2013.

Tuckett, A. G. (2005). Residents' Rights and Nurses Ethics in the Australian Nursing Home. International Nursing Review pp. 52 (3) pp. 219–224.

Tuckett, A. G. (2006). On Paternalism, Autonomy and Best Interests: Telling The (Competent) Aged-Care Resident What they Want To Know. International Journal of Nursing Practice (12) pp. 166–173.

Tuckett, A. G.(2007). The Meaning Of Nursing Home: 'Waiting To Go Up To St.Peter, OK! Waiting House, Sad But True' – An Australian Perspective. Journal Of Aging Studies (21) pp. 119–133.

Tulloch, G. J. (1975). A Home Is Not A Home (Living Within A Nursing Home). New York. The Seaburg Press.

UNISON (2012). Care In The Balance. A UNISON Survey Into Staff/Patient Ratios On Our Wards. Web: unison.org.uk. 1 February 2013.

Vail, D. J. (1996). Dehumanisation and The Institutional Career. USA. Charles Thomas.

Vladeck, C. (1980). Unloving Care. New York. Basic Books.

Vladeck, B. C. (2003). Unloving Care Revisited: The Persistence Of Culture. Journal of Social Work in Longterm Care (2) 1. pp. 1–19.

Voldberg, P. (nd) How Do I Complain About A Skilled Nursing Home Facility? Web: ehow.com/healthcare. 1 February 2013.

Wade, B. Sawyer, L. Bell, J. (1983). Dependency With Dignity. London. Bedford Square Press.

Wallston, K. A. Wallston, B. S. DeVellis, B. M.(1976). Effect of a Negative Stereotype On Nurses' Attitudes Toward an Alcoholic Patient. Journal of Studies in Alcohol v. 37 n. 5 pp. 659–665.

Wells, T. J. (1980). Problems in Geriatric Nursing Care. Churchill Livingstone.

Weiner, J. M. Tilly, J. Howe, A. Doyle, C. Evans Cuellar, A. Campbell, J. Ikegami, N. (2007). Quality Assurance for Long Term Care; The Experiences of England, Australia, Germany and Japan. Web: assets.carp.org/rgcenter/i/2007. 2 February 2013.

Western, M. Baxter, J. Pakulski, J. Tranter, B. Western, J. van Egmond, M. Chesters, J.Hosking, A. O'Flaherty, M. Van Gellecum, Y. (2007). Neoliberalism, inequality and politics: The changing face of Australia. Australian Journal of Social Issues 42 (3) pp. 401–418.

WHO (1994). A Declaration On The Promotion Of Patients' Rights In Europe. Web: who.int/genomics 1 March 2013.

Whiteford, P. (2012). How Far is Australia's Welfare State? Web: Inside.org.uk. 11 June 2012.

Wighton, K. (2011). Nurses Who Laugh at Patients. Drs Who Snub Worried Relatives. And NHS Bosses Who Say manners are a Luxury We Can't Afford': The Rudest hospitals in Britain. Web: mailonline 8 November 2011.

Wikinvest. Web: wikinvest.com. 2 February 2013.

Wilkinson, J. Brittman, M. (2003). Relatives, Friends and Strangers: The Links Between Voluntary Activity, Sociability and Care. Social Policy Research Centre discussion paper n. 125. Web: sprc.unsw.ed.au/media. 2 March 2013.

Williams, D. (2011). Student Nurses Removed From Hospital Amid CQC Concerns. Health service Journal 29 July 2011.

Williams, Z. (2013). Charities' Silence On Government Policy is Tantamount To Collusion. Web: guardian.co.uk. 22 January 2013.

Woogara, J. (2005). Patients' Privacy Of The Person and Human Rights. Nursing Ethics 12 (3) pp. 273–287.

Wright, S. (2001). Nursing Development Units: Progress and Developments Nursing Standard, 15 (29) pp. 39–41 22 November 2001.

Wrigley, T. (2008). Educationalfutures v. 1 (2) December 2008.

Ziegenfuss, J. T. (2010). The Ombudsman Handbook: Designing and Managing an Effective Problem-Solving Programme Web: books.google.co.uk. 1 April 2013.

Image References

All images by Keiren Robertshaw (Graphic Designer).

WHO OWNS CARE HOMES?

Lenin Nightingale

Care Homes in the UK are increasingly being controlled by private equity businesses, as witnessed by the acquisition of Four Seasons Health Care by Terra Firma, a private equity group which agreed a £825m takeover. Four Seasons had debts which totalled £1.6bn in 2009. The Royal Bank of Scotland took a 40% stake in the company in return for nearly halving its debt. .(bbc.co.uk2012)

Acting on behalf of pension funds, insurance companies, and rich clients, private equity groups manage companies on behalf of their investors.

Why should nurses, patients' relatives, and the taxpayer be concerned by such developments? After all, the world of high finance does not claim the interest of many, as it is seen as the perogative of highly educated 'city types' who can grasp its perplexing intricacies.

Firstly, then, allow me to put in simple terms what it is that private equity businesses do:

They acquire a controlling interest in companies with a *large proportion of debt* relative to equity. The acquisition is leveraged, that is, it is financed by borrowing money against the acquired company's assets and future stock market performance.

The aim is to *increase the stock market value of the company* by hoping the market reacts positively to changes in management, which are often accompanied by bullish statements about future performances. When Terra Firma acquired EMI in 2007, it issued statements about its troubled past and better future: EMI lacked "business discipline", and wise investors would appreciate "the significant potential for transforming the business". Compare this with this statement by Peter Calveley, CEO of 'Four Seasons', "We have now got in place a stable long-term capital structure that means we have got confidence in our position". (Brindle, 2012). This came after 'Four Seasons' was acquired by Terra Firma in a £825m. deal underwritten by Barclays and Goldman Sachs. £700m was in the form of loans, and the balance of £125m was raised from investors. In the 'Four Seasons' example, if its stock market value increased to £1bn., the return to investors will be £1bn. – £700m., that is, £300m., representing a return on investment of 140%.

This form of speculative business model depends on rising stock markets to enable selling on at a higher valuation - such businesses only buy to sell on. When stock markets are in decline, the exit strategy becomes problematic.

This business model differs from venture capital partnerships that usually invest in start-ups, and do not take a controlling interest in the acquired company. The *speculative* model distributes cash generated by the acquired company to investors on a contractual basis, that is, they do not act like the majority of companies, which pay discretionary dividends. The *speculators* also charge a per annum management fee, usually of between 2-3%. They can also claim a share of profits when the company is sold; in the above example, this could be as much as 20% of the £300m 'profit'.

This business model relies on the availability of cheap and 'flexible' borrowing, with interest paid *flexibly* during the term of the loan. Banks securitize their lending, so that it does not appear on their balance sheet, which increases their ability to lend more. Loans can be on very 'easy' terms, often with clauses that allow default on repayment at least once without incurring penalty.

It is a vast commission generating merry-go-round in which the elderly have become a commodity.

What's more, it is speculation that cannot fail; consider the case of Southern Cross, which the private equity firm Blackstone bought for £162million in 2004, selling it three years later at considerable profit, which it achieved by selling off the company's homes (45 to 'Four Seasons'), and forcing Southern Cross to lease the properties back. This arrangement contributed to Southern Cross going into administration, with the government immediately pledging to use public money to ensure affected homes would stay open, amid warnings that moving vulnerable patients might lead to their deaths. It is like going into a bookmakers and placing a bet than cannot lose; the tax payer will return all losing stakes. 'Four Seasons' eventually acquired (by debt finance)140 care homes from Southern Cross.

The private equity model (scam) borrows at high levels using the asset they're seeking to acquire as collateral on the debt; indebt the company further on the promise of 'performance improvements,' pay off their major creditors, and relying on the tax payer to pick up the bill. In the case of 'Four Seasons', this increased indebtedness is underway, it acquiring 17 care homes from Optimum Care, which operated under the Avery banner, owned by Graphite Capital, another private equity investor (healthinvestor.co.uk 11 April 2013).

Investment banking revenues increase from underwriting private equity debt finance and charging fees for setting up deals, but the mechanics of these deals can easily collapse. As private equity partners face debt repayment deadlines they may need to sell parts of their investment, or seek re-financing deals at higher cost to finance existing debt.

What of the quality of care provided under the aegis of such companies. "Helga Pile, Unison national officer for social services, said: "Private Equity takeovers are noted for looking at ways of maximising profits. The elderly care sector by contrast is woefully underfunded and cannot afford to lower the quality of care by cutting staff or depressing the training and wages of people who work in it." (bbc.co.uk 30 April 2012). Regarding the training and wages of workers, Peter Calveley lamented that 'Four Seasons' needed to recruit "several hundred" nurses from elsewhere in the EU, principally Spain, Portugal and Romania (Brindle, 2012).

They are mainly what are described as PRN nurses, that is, qualified nurses currently undergoing NMC registration, who can be employed as nurses, but who will start off as senior nursing assistants or senior carers while waiting for their registration to be completed. These nurses need to apply for an accession card which ties them to their employer. "Romanian and Bulgarian immigrant workers might be unwanted by the British public, but they are in high demand from British employers, with almost 48,000 UK jobs offered on a careers website in Romania last year. Recruitment agent Brindusa Deac, of Tjobs, Romanias largest foreign jobs website, said: "I don't think an employer in Britain minds what nationality they employ, they want the best candidate for the *cheapest wage legally possible*. And Romanians will *probably earn less* than a Briton in the same position. Around 40% of the jobs offered on the website are for healthcare staff, most for elderly careworkers for both private and state-run care homes. The government has confirmed it will not seek to extend temporary curbs on 29 million Romanian and Bulgarian nationals' right to live and work in Britain, which are due to expire in December" (Elgot, 2013).

Many of these workers are offered accommodation by their employee, often within or attached to the place of work, for which they are charged, and are on-call at all times, with nurses often being asked to cover for ill carers. Of care assistants: "These are hard working reliable individuals looking for work as a carer, they may *not have care experience* but will undergo *the normal 2–5 days training* as required by care home providers. While these positions are mainly live out, employers who do not have staff accommodation are expected to help migrant staff to find suitable cheap rooms in the local area and possibly cover the first few weeks rent for them until they start getting paid (easterneuropeans.co.uk 2013). Yet the CQC requirement in England is for a course based on *Skills For Care*. The duration of this course and its exact content is not specified, and it is assessed by the registered manager of the establishment .

It is within this business model that: "UNISON has reached a landmark recognition agreement with Four Seasons Health Care along with the GMB and the Royal College of Nursing" (unison.org.uk 5 February 2013). Perhaps this statement by the RCN may summarise what use the unions can be to 'Four Seasons' – "we can help you to achieve your *business objectives*" (rcn.org.uk February 2012).Surely a role of any Union is to support members when raising issues of patient care in addition to supporting demands for greater pay and conditions- which would fly against the business objectives actually.

Why does it not matter that newly qualified UK nurses are not being recruited in sufficient numbers into the private care home sector? The answer: because they will never be able to compete in terms of cost and 'flexibility' with EU nationals, and this is a portent of what will become the guiding principle of all areas of nursing within the UK. Nurses face the same prospect as call centre workers, whose jobs went to areas of low labour cost.

Nurses, like Boxer, the workhorse in George Orwell's Animal Farm, described as the farm's most dedicated and loyal labourer, are being sent to the knackers' yard in a van owned by private equity firms and driven by unions. The £15bn care-for-the-elderly market is expected to grow at 3.1% a year for the next 10 years. Everyone wants to be a part of it. "Finding out who owns a nursing home should be easy. According to a new Government Accountability Office report, it's not. Private investment firms have been buying up nursing homes in recent years, creating a complicated trail that makes ownership difficult to pinpoint. This lack of transparency makes it difficult to know who is ultimately responsible for care in a home" (desmoinesregister 2013).

References

Bbc.co.uk (20120
Terra Firma To Buy Four Seasons Healthcare for £825m
Bbc.co.uk/news 30.4
Brindle D (2012)
Peter Calveley of Four Seasons Healthcare; 'I Can See A Lot of Pain'
The Guardian 11.12
Desmoinesregster.com
Make it Clear Who Owns Nursing Homes 1.11
Elgot J (2013)
Romanian Immigrants Have 'Pick Of Thousands of UK Jobs' Recruiter Says
The Huffington Post 28.1
Health Investor.co.uk (2013)
Fshc.co.uk
Company News 11.4

CPSIA information can be obtained
at www.ICGtesting.com
Printed in the USA
LVOW04s0117051215

465434LV00017B/708/P